Medication

Calculations

IT'S EASIER THAN YOU THINK

Medication Calculations

IT'S EASIER THAN YOU THINK

Kim Leong

MA, RN, CNT, Cert. Ed., NT

Senior Lecturer in Nursing Studies, University of Cumbria, Lancaster Campus

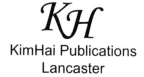

KimHai Publications

Lancaster

© 2008 KimHai Publications Lancaster

First published in 2008 by KimHai Publications
18, Highgrove Road,
Lancaster,
Lancashire,
England,
LA1 5FS

British Library Cataloguing in Publication Data

A catalogue record for this book is available from the British Library

ISBN 978-0-9553797-1-0

Printed and bound by Athenaeum Press Limited, Dukesway, Team Valley, Gateshead, Tyne and Wear, NE11 0PZ. Email: www.athenaeumpress.co.uk.

Medication Calculations
It's easier than you think!

'This book should be of use to nurses and other healthcare professionals needing to learn or refresh their numeracy skills. The book splits things up into easy to follow chapters with a full range of questions and answers to help grasp the subject of drug calculations.'

Mark Magas BPharm, MRPharmS

CONTENTS

Forward ix

Acknowledgements xi

Chapter 1
Units of measurement: Weight, Volume and Distance

Standard symbol for measurement 1

Chapter 2
Decimals, Fractions and Percentages 5

Chapter 3
Conversion of metric weights 25

Chapter 4
Conversion of metric volumes 31

Chapter 5
Calculate drug dosages accurately by using a formula 35

Chapter 6
Calculate the infusion flow rate for blood and fluids by using a formula 41

Chapter 7
Calculate the flow rate for a drug in an infusion fluid 47

Chapter 8
Ratios and Percentages 53

Chapter 9

Calculate Paediatric dosages 57

Chapter 10

Calculate the correct dosages when using a syringe driver to

administer drugs 63

Chapter 11

Understand the law when dealing with medications 67

Chapter 12

Why tablets should not be crushed and capsules should not be opened 73

Chapter 13

Descriptive statistics 77

Index 93

FORWARD

For the past three decades nurses have been taught how to organise their patient care based on a problem-solving approach and yet there has not been a book published to guide them in working out drug dosages based on this problem-solving approach.

This book is a manual to encourage this approach. It has been developed as a result of a research project carried out by the author in 1993 on sixty-nine "Project 2,000 student nurses" and first-hand experience teaching on Intravenous Workshops for qualified nurses from 1994 to 2001.

The drive towards a problem-solving approach will not only enhance nurses' calculating skills but also enable them to relate to their every day drug administration. The intention, therefore, is to support nurses who want to perfect their skills in drug calculations in order to prevent any mistakes, which can cost lives. Since there is no substitute for "understanding", this book is intended to equip nurses with the understanding necessary to make accurate calculations.

To build your confidence, this book will begin with a review of basic mathematics. It includes: - units of measurement, decimals, multiplication and division of fractions, ratios, proportions and percentages. Revision exercises (answers are provided at the back of this book) have been added at the end of chapter two in order to assist you to revise your understanding each concept. (The understanding of these concepts is essential for accurate calculation of drug dosages later on).

This will be followed by real life drug calculations. Each chapter will begin by showing mistakes (in calculation) commonly made by some nurses. Reasons for these mistakes will be highlighted, followed by a step-by-step explanation of how to avoid similar mistakes. Specific medications and realistic drug calculations are used throughout for the sake of authenticity. The reader is then invited to complete some practice examples (answers are provided at the back of this book).

ACKNOWLEDGEMENTS

I would like to thank my wife for continuing patience, encouragement and support.

I would like to thank my children, Mei Ling, Mei Yee and Kim Ming for ideas for the book cover, illustrations and proof-reading and last but not least my youngest son, Kim Wai for just pure inspiration! I would also like to thank my niece Hannah Gosling for help with the chapter on Fractions and Ratios.

Finally, a special thanks to Mark Magas who has done the entire checking, proof reading and assisted with editing the book.

CHAPTER ONE

> **Learning Outcomes**
>
> At the end of this chapter, you will be able to understand: -
> - ❖ Units of measurement
> - ❖ Weight, Volume and Distance
> - ❖ Standard symbol for measurement

(A) The United Kingdom originally used the Imperial system of measurement in which the common units were: -

Weight: ounce, pound, stone, hundredweight, ton
Volume: gill, pint, quart, gallon
Distance: inch, foot, yard, mile

From the 1960s onwards all educational institutions have used the S.I. (Système Internationale) or metric system as used throughout the mainland Europe. This system uses the following Units: -

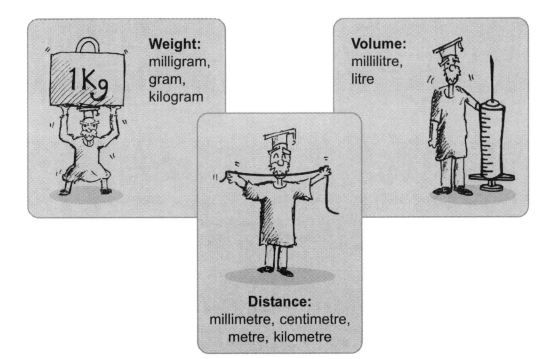

Weight: milligram, gram, kilogram

Volume: millilitre, litre

Distance: millimetre, centimetre, metre, kilometre

Unlike decimalisation of the currency, which took place on a single day in 1971, there has been a gradual changeover from imperial to metric, largely on an industry-by-industry basis. For example the construction industry changed over in the 1970s but the labelling of goods for the food and drink industry has only taken place in the 1990s. Some Imperial measurements are still in common use and likely to remain that way e.g. the mile for transport purposes.

In the Health Service, prescriptions and dosages are all given in metric units.

(B) The standard metric units for weight, volume and distance were mentioned earlier. You can see a common format: -

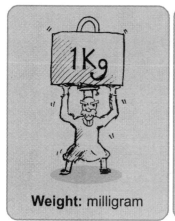
Weight: milligram

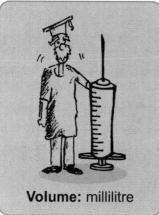
Volume: millilitre

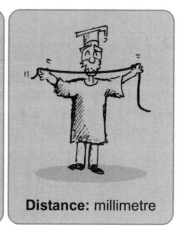
Distance: millimetre

milli... means 'one thousandth part of'   =   **÷ 1000**

kilo.... means 'one thousand times bigger than'   =   **x 1000**

1 milligram is therefore one-thousandth part of a gram and is a small quantity.

1 kilogram, on the other hand, is one thousand times bigger than a gram and is therefore a large quantity.

Standard symbols are used as abbreviations for units:

gram	=	g	milligram	=	mg	kilogram	=	kg
litre	=	l	millilitre	=	ml			
metre	=	m	millimetre	=	mm	kilometre	=	km

(C) The metric system has been used throughout the hospitals in the United Kingdom since 1975. Because dosages can involve very small quantities, an even smaller weight than a milligram is frequently used. This smaller weight is called a microgram. Micro means one-millionth part of so that there are 1,000,000 micrograms in 1 gram.

The <u>standard</u> symbol for microgram is µg (µ being a Greek letter, pronounced *mew*). However, when prescriptions are written by hand it is extremely easy to confuse µ with m. For this reason the Health Service uses a <u>non-standard</u> symbol for microgram, mcg, which avoids the confusion.

The relative sizes of the units can now be expressed as, for example:

$1 \text{ g} = 1\ 000 \text{ mg}$ $1 \text{ g} = 1\ 000\ 000 \text{ mcg}$ $1 \text{ mg} = 1\ 000 \text{ mcg}$

$1 \text{ mg} = \dfrac{1}{1\ 000} \text{ g}$ $1 \text{ mcg} = \dfrac{1}{1\ 000} \text{ mg}$ $1 \text{ mcg} = \dfrac{1}{1\ 000\ 000} \text{ g}$

(D) Light objects, such as medicines, are usually measured in grams, kilograms, milligrams or micrograms. However, heavier weights, like babies, infants and adults, are measured in pounds (lb) and kilograms (kg). Imperial units of measurement such as pounds (lb) and ounces (oz) are still used in some wards.

To change pounds into kilograms, you divide by 2.2
To change kilograms into pounds, you multiply by 2.2

Exercise 1

1)	4.4 lb	=	kg	6)	33 lb	=	kg
2)	19.8 lb	=	kg	7)	132 lb	=	kg
3)	50.6 lb	=	kg	8)	88 lb	=	kg
4)	13.2 lb	=	kg	9)	11 lb	=	kg
5)	6.6 lb	=	kg	10)	15.4 lb	=	kg

Remember

To change pounds into kilograms, you divide by 2.2
To change kilograms into pounds, you multiply by 2.2

Exercise 1 (continued)

11) 4 kg = lb	16) 10 kg = lb
12) 2 kg = lb	17) 45 kg = lb
13) 5.5 kg = lb	18) 8.8 kg = lb
14) 6.2 kg = lb	19) 35 kg = lb
15) 7.6 kg = lb	20) 11.1 kg = lb

Summary – Units of Measurement

1 kilogram	1000 grams
1 gram	1000 milligrams
1 milligram	1000 micrograms
1 kilogram	2.2 pounds
1 litre	1000 millilitres
1 kilometre	1000 metres
1 metre	100 centimetres
1 centimetre	10 millimetres

CHAPTER TWO

Learning Outcomes

At the end of this chapter, you will be able to understand: -

❖ What decimals are
❖ What fractions are
❖ What percentages are
❖ What ratios are
❖ How to multiply a number by 10, 100 and 1000
❖ How to divide a number by 10, 100 and 1000
❖ How to multiply a fraction by a whole number
❖ How to turn improper fractions into mixed fractions
❖ How to reduce fractions to their simplest form
❖ How to convert fractions into percentages and vice versa

Basic Arithmetic
Converting decimals

To multiply a decimal by 10, 100, and 1000, all you have to do is move the decimal point.

E.g. the decimal 0.1

0.1 x 10 = 1 Since there is only one 0 (zero) in the 10, you move the decimal point one place to the right.

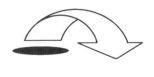

0.1 x 100 = 10 Since there are two 0's (zeros) in the 100, you move the decimal point two places to the right.

 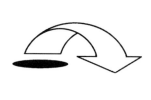 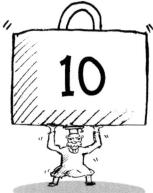

0.1 x 1000 = 100 Since there are three 0's (zeros) in 1000, you move the decimal point three places to the right.

 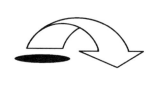 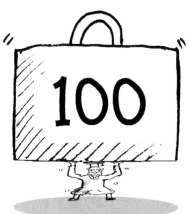

Exercise 1

Multiplication of a decimal by 10, 100, 1000

Example

0.46 x 100 Move the decimal point two places to the right = 46

Without using a calculator, find out the value of:

1) 0.35 x 10 =	4) 0.99 x 10 =	7) 4.6 x 10 =
2) 0.71 x 100 =	5) 0.52 x 100 =	8) 8.5 x 100 =
3) 0.2 x 1000 =	6) 1.2 x 1000 =	9) 6.7 x 1000 =

Exercise 1 (continued)

10) 4.617238 x 10 =

11) 1.6 x 100 =

12) 0.32 x 10 =

13) 0.28 x 1000 =

14) 6.8 x 1000 =

15) 0.078 x 100 =

16) 13.3 x 100 =

17) 14.7 x 10 =

18) 0.55 x 10 =

19) 0.018 x 10 =

20) 0.034 x 1000 =

21) 0.212 x 10 =

22) 7.25 x 100 =

23) 0.14 x 1000 =

24) 0.0295 x 100 =

25) 0.178 x 10 =

26) 88.12 x 100 =

27) 6.012 x 1000 =

28) 0.0041 x 100 =

29) 6.72 x 100 =

30) 9.01 x 10 =

31) 0.09 x 1000 =

32) 8.701 x 10 =

33) 1.001 x 100 =

34) 0.805 x 10 =

35) 9.9 x 100 =

36) 6.67 x 1000 =

37) 5.051 x 100 =

38) 10.99 x 10 =

39) 8.011 x 100 =

40) 9.911 x 1000 =

Summary

Multiplication by (number)	Numberof zeros	Move the decimal point (to the right)
10	1	1 place
100	2	2 places
1000	3	3 places

To divide a decimal by 10, 100, or 1000, you also only have to move the decimal point.

E.g. the decimal 0.1

0.1 ÷ 10 = 0.01 this time, instead of moving the decimal point to the right, you move it to the left 1 place as there is only one 0 (zero) in 10.

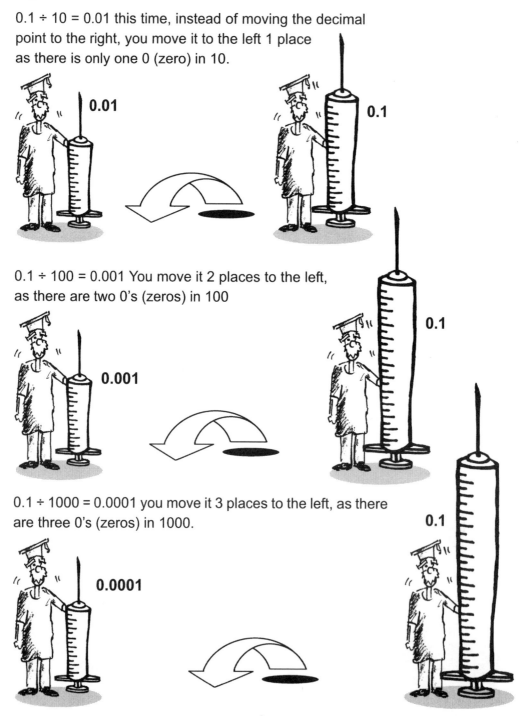

0.1 ÷ 100 = 0.001 You move it 2 places to the left, as there are two 0's (zeros) in 100

0.1 ÷ 1000 = 0.0001 you move it 3 places to the left, as there are three 0's (zeros) in 1000.

Exercise 2

Division of a decimal by 10, 100, 1000

Example

$46 \div 100$ Move the decimal point two places to the left $= 0.46$

Without using a calculator, find out the value of:

1) $0.7 \div 10 =$

2) $0.62 \div 100 =$

3) $0.95 \div 100 =$

4) $0.11 \div 1000 =$

5) $0.78 \div 10000 =$

6) $1.45 \div 100 =$

7) $10.7 \div 10 =$

8) $100.56 \div 1000 =$

9) $56.73 \div 100 =$

10) $701.2 \div 1000 =$

11) $75.38 \div 10 =$

12) $0.068 \div 100 =$

13) $15.8 \div 10 =$

14) $0.87 \div 10 =$

15) $0.45 \div 100 =$

16) $0.78 \div 1000 =$

17) $5.9 \div 100 =$

18) $426 \div 100 =$

19) $188.5 \div 100 =$

20) $17.9 \div 1000 =$

21) $0.09 \div 10 =$

22) $0.71 \div 100 =$

23) $0.091 \div 10 =$

24) $993.1 \div 100 =$

25) $80.31 \div 100 =$

26) $99.51 \div 1000 =$

27) $101.1 \div 10 =$

28) $669.1 \div 100 =$

29) $10.101 \div 10 =$

30) $876.1 \div 100 =$

31) $991.1 \div 100 =$

32) $41.3 \div 100 =$

33) $83.41 \div 1000 =$

34) $6.011 \div 10 =$

35) $73.05 \div 10 =$

36) $0.951 \div 10 =$

37) $443.1 \div 100 =$

38) $6.91 \div 100 =$

39) $340.1 \div 10 =$

40) $91.09 \div 1000 =$

Summary

Division by (number)	Numberof zeros	Move the decimal point (to the left)
10	1	1 place
100	2	2 places
1000	3	3 places

Fractions

What is a fraction?

A fraction is a mathematical expression for a part(s) of a whole or one number divided by another number. In any fraction, the number above the dividing line is called the numerator. It represents the number of part(s) of the whole. The number below the dividing line is called the denominator, and it represents the number of parts into which the whole is divided.

A whole is split into equal parts.

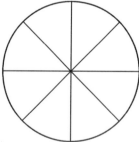

For example, let's say the following cake is a whole.

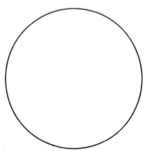

A fraction, $\frac{1}{2}$ means that 1 whole is divided into 2 equal parts and that only 1 part of the 2 parts is being used. In the following illustration, the shaded area is equal to $\frac{1}{2}$.

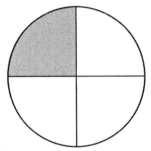

Similarly, $\frac{1}{4}$ means that the whole is divided into 4 equal parts and that 1 part of the 4 parts is being used.

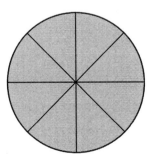

A fraction that has the same numerator and denominator always equals to 1. For example, the fraction $\frac{8}{8}$ means that the whole number 1 has been divided into 8 equal parts, and all parts are being used.

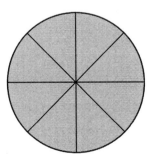

The larger the denominator, the greater is the number of equal parts. For example, in this fraction $\frac{1}{4}$, the '4' indicates that the whole number has been divided into 4 equal parts. In the fraction $\frac{1}{8}$, the denominator indicates that the whole number has been divided into 8 equal parts. Therefore, as the denominator becomes larger, the size of the parts becomes smaller. So, $\frac{1}{4}$ is bigger than $\frac{1}{8}$.

What Are Equivalent Fractions?

Even though equivalent fractions look different, they are actually **equal in value**. They must have the same 'multiplier' **top** (numerator) and **bottom** (denominator). Think of any fraction you like, and make up a list of equivalent fractions by simply multiplying the numerator and denominator by the same number each time, as shown below:

$$\frac{1}{2} = \frac{2}{4} = \frac{3}{6} = \frac{4}{8} = \frac{5}{10} = \frac{6}{12} = \frac{\text{any number}}{\textbf{TWICE that number}}$$

$$\frac{1}{4} = \frac{2}{8} = \frac{3}{12} = \frac{4}{16} = \frac{5}{20} = \frac{6}{24} = \frac{\text{any number}}{\textbf{FOUR TIMES that number}}$$

Exercise 3

Example

$$\frac{1}{2} = \frac{}{4} = \frac{3}{8} = \frac{}{8} = \frac{5}{12} = \frac{}{12} = \frac{1}{2} = \frac{2}{4} = \frac{3}{6} = \frac{4}{8} = \frac{5}{10} = \frac{6}{12}$$

Fill in the blanks for these following equivalent fractions:

1) $\dfrac{1}{3} = \dfrac{}{6} = \dfrac{3}{12} = \dfrac{5}{} = \dfrac{}{18}$

2) $\dfrac{1}{5} = \dfrac{2}{} = \dfrac{}{15} = \dfrac{4}{25} = \dfrac{6}{}$

3) $\dfrac{1}{8} = \dfrac{}{16} = \dfrac{3}{32} = \dfrac{5}{} = \dfrac{}{48}$

4) $\dfrac{1}{7} = \dfrac{2}{} = \dfrac{}{21} = \dfrac{4}{35} = \dfrac{6}{}$

5) $\dfrac{1}{9} = \dfrac{}{18} = \dfrac{3}{} = \dfrac{}{36} = \dfrac{5}{54}$

Going the other way, you will sometimes need to **simplify** by 'cancelling down' - this means dividing the numerator and denominator by the same number:

$$\frac{3}{9} = \frac{\div 3}{\div 3} = \frac{1}{3}$$

$$\frac{11}{44} = \frac{\div 11}{\div 11} = \frac{1}{4}$$

Exercise 4

Example

$$\frac{24}{48} = \frac{12}{24} = \frac{6}{12} = \frac{3}{6} = \frac{1}{2}$$

Simplify the following fractions to their lowest terms:

1) $\dfrac{2}{4} =$

2) $\dfrac{3}{15} =$

3) $\dfrac{8}{32} =$

4) $\dfrac{11}{99} =$

5) $\dfrac{54}{63} =$

6) $\dfrac{6}{12} =$

7) $\dfrac{7}{28} =$

8) $\dfrac{9}{72} =$

9) $\dfrac{24}{36} =$

10) $\dfrac{5}{35} =$

11) $\dfrac{12}{16} =$

12) $\dfrac{10}{50} =$

13) $\dfrac{42}{56} =$

14) $\dfrac{14}{49} =$

15) $\dfrac{25}{30} =$

16) $\dfrac{80}{100} =$

17) $\dfrac{5}{20} =$

18) $\dfrac{24}{42} =$

19) $\dfrac{18}{39} =$

20) $\dfrac{22}{66} =$

21) $\dfrac{60}{120} =$

22) $\dfrac{27}{81} =$

23) $\dfrac{10}{35} =$

24) $\dfrac{8}{28} =$

25) $\dfrac{48}{108} =$

26) $\dfrac{5}{15} =$

27) $\dfrac{2}{26} =$

28) $\dfrac{33}{132} =$

29) $\dfrac{90}{100} =$

30) $\dfrac{8}{44} =$

31) $\dfrac{28}{35} =$

32) $\dfrac{10}{95} =$

33) $\dfrac{25}{100} =$

34) $\dfrac{48}{56} =$

35) $\dfrac{7}{105} =$

36) $\dfrac{54}{99} =$

37) $\dfrac{12}{81} =$

38) $\dfrac{58}{92} =$

39) $\dfrac{55}{99} =$

40) $\dfrac{21}{63} =$

Multiplication of fractions

To multiply a fraction by a whole number is multiplying two fractions with the second fraction (which is the whole number) always having a one in the denominator.

Example 1

Whole number

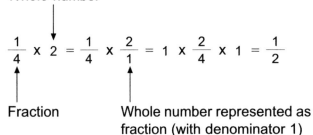

Fraction   Whole number represented as fraction (with denominator 1)

Example 2

Whole number

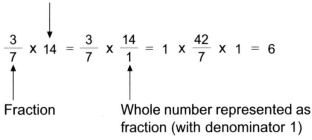

Fraction   Whole number represented as fraction (with denominator 1)

Exercise 5

Multiplication of a fraction by a whole number

Find out the values of:

1) $\dfrac{1}{3}$ x 3 =

2) $\dfrac{1}{2}$ x 5 =

3) $\dfrac{1}{7}$ x 4 =

4) $\dfrac{1}{5}$ x 6 =

5) $\dfrac{1}{6}$ x 2 =

6) $\dfrac{2}{3}$ x 7 =

7) $\dfrac{2}{2}$ x 3 =

8) $\dfrac{2}{4}$ x 5 =

9) $\dfrac{2}{7}$ x 9 =

10) $\dfrac{2}{9}$ x 4 =

11) $\dfrac{3}{4}$ x 2 =

12) $\dfrac{3}{7}$ x 3 =

Exercise 5 (continued)

13) $\dfrac{3}{10}$ x 5 =

14) $\dfrac{3}{8}$ x 7 =

15) $\dfrac{3}{14}$ x 9 =

16) $\dfrac{4}{4}$ x 2 =

17) $\dfrac{4}{9}$ x 4 =

18) $\dfrac{4}{14}$ x 12 =

19) $\dfrac{4}{6}$ x 7 =

20) $\dfrac{4}{10}$ x 9 =

21) $\dfrac{5}{7}$ x 5 =

22) $\dfrac{5}{6}$ x 9 =

23) $\dfrac{5}{14}$ x 3 =

24) $\dfrac{5}{21}$ x 11 =

25) $\dfrac{5}{9}$ x 10 =

26) $\dfrac{6}{7}$ x 4 =

27) $\dfrac{6}{9}$ x 7 =

28) $\dfrac{6}{58}$ x 5 =

29) $\dfrac{6}{22}$ x 3 =

30) $\dfrac{7}{9}$ x 2 =

31) $\dfrac{7}{10}$ x 7 =

32) $\dfrac{7}{15}$ x 8 =

33) $\dfrac{7}{19}$ x 2 =

34) $\dfrac{7}{8}$ x 4 =

35) $\dfrac{8}{10}$ x 5 =

36) $\dfrac{8}{12}$ x 2 =

37) $\dfrac{9}{11}$ x 3 =

38) $\dfrac{9}{14}$ x 4 =

39) $\dfrac{9}{15}$ x 6 =

40) $\dfrac{9}{15}$ x 7 =

A mixed fraction is one that contains both a whole number and a fractione.g. $1\frac{1}{4}$.

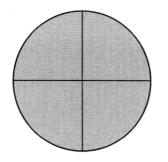 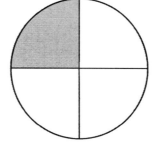

Whole number
(1 in this case)

$+$

Fraction
($\frac{1}{4}$ in this case)

An improper fraction is a fraction in which the numerator is larger than the denominator, resulting in a number greater than one e.g. $\frac{5}{4}$.

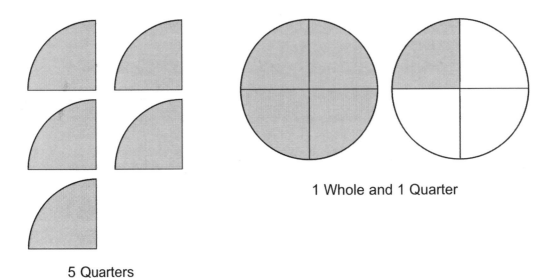

1 Whole and 1 Quarter

5 Quarters

How to turn improper fractions into mixed fractions

To turn this improper fraction into a mixed fraction, you do as follows:

Divide 37 by 8, giving a whole number of 4 and a remainder of 5.

The remainder then becomes the numerator, in this case 5. The denominator, 8, is kept the same, so the remainder fraction is $\frac{5}{8}$.

Put them together and the answer becomes a mixed number, $4\frac{5}{8}$.

Exercise 6

Converting improper fractions into mixed fractions.

Find out the values of:

1) $\dfrac{9}{4} =$ 5) $\dfrac{88}{9} =$ 9) $\dfrac{49}{10} =$ 13) $\dfrac{41}{3} =$

2) $\dfrac{17}{4} =$ 6) $\dfrac{9}{2} =$ 10) $\dfrac{7}{2} =$ 14) $\dfrac{83}{7} =$

3) $\dfrac{37}{6} =$ 7) $\dfrac{15}{4} =$ 11) $\dfrac{91}{8} =$ 15) $\dfrac{127}{5} =$

4) $\dfrac{53}{10} =$ 8) $\dfrac{91}{6} =$ 12) $\dfrac{27}{4} =$ 16) $\dfrac{41}{8} =$

Exercise 6 (continued)

17) $\dfrac{67}{5} =$

18) $\dfrac{115}{11} =$

19) $\dfrac{15}{6} =$

20) $\dfrac{11}{3} =$

21) $\dfrac{77}{5} =$

22) $\dfrac{5}{4} =$

23) $\dfrac{72}{9} =$

24) $\dfrac{10}{6} =$

25) $\dfrac{33}{2} =$

26) $\dfrac{54}{9} =$

27) $\dfrac{92}{15} =$

28) $\dfrac{42}{9} =$

29) $\dfrac{65}{10} =$

30) $\dfrac{15}{14} =$

31) $\dfrac{24}{16} =$

32) $\dfrac{77}{6} =$

33) $\dfrac{35}{14} =$

34) $\dfrac{14}{9} =$

35) $\dfrac{27}{22} =$

36) $\dfrac{91}{52} =$

37) $\dfrac{13}{7} =$

38) $\dfrac{5}{3} =$

39) $\dfrac{111}{81} =$

40) $\dfrac{67}{3} =$

How to reduce improper fractions to their simplest form

Fractions in which the same number can divide both the numerator and the denominator can be reduced to a simpler form, for example $\dfrac{10}{28}$,

How do we reduce $\dfrac{10}{28}$ to its lowest terms? Like this:

Take the fraction $\dfrac{10}{28}$. Find the lowest **common factor** of 10 and 28, which is 2, in this case.

Divide the numerator and denominator by the common factor.

$$\dfrac{10}{28} = \dfrac{10 \div 2}{28 \div 2} = \dfrac{5}{14}$$

Exercise 7

Reducing improper fractions to their simplest forms

Simplify these fractions into their lowest forms:

1) $\dfrac{12}{16} =$

2) $\dfrac{2}{4} =$

3) $\dfrac{6}{12} =$

4) $\dfrac{10}{50} =$

5) $\dfrac{42}{56} =$

6) $\dfrac{48}{36} =$

7) $\dfrac{14}{49} =$

8) $\dfrac{28}{7} =$

9) $\dfrac{25}{30} =$

10) $\dfrac{100}{80} =$

11) $\dfrac{5}{20} =$

12) $\dfrac{24}{42} =$

13) $\frac{39}{19}$ =

14) $\frac{22}{66}$ =

15) $\frac{60}{120}$ =

16) $\frac{27}{81}$ =

17) $\frac{35}{10}$ =

18) $\frac{8}{28}$ =

19) $\frac{3}{6}$ =

20) $\frac{48}{108}$ =

What is a percentage?

A percentage is another way of expressing a fraction in which the denominator is 100, for example if you divided a cake into 100 equal portions, each portion would be the fraction $\frac{1}{100}$ of the whole cake. This fraction, $\frac{1}{100}$, is called 1 percent, written as 1%. Three portions, $\frac{3}{100}$ is 3%; fifty seven portions, $\frac{57}{100}$ is 57%.

Here are some other percentages: 50%, 40%, 72%, 96%, 200%, 107%, 14%, 23.1%, 81.29%, 315.8%, 0.2%

Converting fractions into percentages

To convert a fraction into a percentage, you have to multiply the fraction by 100%, like this sum:

$\frac{1}{4}$ x 100% then, the sum turns into this:

$\frac{1}{4}$ x $\frac{100}{1}$ = $\frac{100}{4}$ then, you simplify it so the answer is 25%.

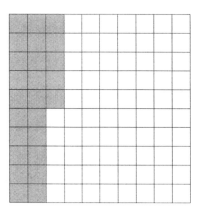

The large square has 100 small squares. 25 small squares are shaded. 25 out of 100, is the fraction $\frac{25}{100}$. 25 out of 100 is 25%.

Exercise 8

Converting fractions into percentages

Convert the following fractions into percentages:

1) $\dfrac{1}{20}$ =

2) $\dfrac{1}{10}$ =

3) $\dfrac{1}{25}$ =

4) $\dfrac{1}{5}$ =

5) $\dfrac{1}{2}$ =

6) $\dfrac{2}{5}$ =

7) $\dfrac{2}{8}$ =

8) $\dfrac{2}{2}$ =

9) $\dfrac{2}{20}$ =

10) $\dfrac{2}{10}$ =

11) $\dfrac{3}{2}$ =

12) $\dfrac{3}{4}$ =

13) $\dfrac{4}{2}$ =

14) $\dfrac{4}{5}$ =

15) $\dfrac{3}{12}$ =

16) $\dfrac{3}{10}$ =

17) $\dfrac{3}{20}$ =

18) $\dfrac{4}{25}$ =

19) $\dfrac{4}{50}$ =

20) $\dfrac{4}{20}$ =

21) $\dfrac{4}{20}$ =

22) $\dfrac{4}{90}$ =

23) $\dfrac{20}{100}$ =

24) $\dfrac{4}{10}$ =

25) $\dfrac{6}{4}$ =

26) $\dfrac{6}{50}$ =

27) $\dfrac{9}{4}$ =

28) $\dfrac{5}{5}$ =

29) $\dfrac{29}{5}$ =

30) $\dfrac{3}{25}$ =

31) $\dfrac{6}{25}$ =

32) $\dfrac{12}{50}$ =

33) $\dfrac{9}{5}$ =

34) $\dfrac{4}{25}$ =

35) $\dfrac{72}{4}$ =

36) $\dfrac{16}{20}$ =

37) $\dfrac{5}{20}$ =

38) $\dfrac{9}{20}$ =

39) $\dfrac{19}{20}$ =

40) $\dfrac{23}{25}$ =

Converting percentages into fractions

To convert a percentage into a fraction, you have to put the percentage as a fraction, with 100 as the denominator.

E.g. 25% you put it over 100, like this

$\dfrac{25}{100}$ and then simplify it.

$$\dfrac{25}{100} = \dfrac{1}{4}$$

Exercise 9

Converting percentages into fractions.

Convert the following percentages into fractions:

1) 13% =	6) 78% =	11) 21% =	16) 93% =
2) 62% =	7) 9% =	12) 201% =	17) 56% =
3) 5% =	8) 48% =	13) 41% =	18) 16% =
4) 71% =	9) 33% =	14) 108% =	19) 110% =
5) 26% =	10) 97% =	15) 55% =	20) 84% =

What is a ratio?

A ratio consists of 2 or more figures that are separated by a colon

E.g. 1:2

A ratio is related to a fraction, and it also has a numerator and denominator.

E.g. 1:2 $= \dfrac{1}{2}$ ←——— numerator
←——— denominator

1:2 means 1 part to 2 parts, just like fractions.

What is a Proportion?

A proportion is a mathematical relation of equality between two ratios, having the form:-

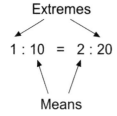

Extremes

1 : 10 = 2 : 20

Means

The inner numbers of the proportion are known as means whereas the outer ones are called extremes. In this proportion, the product of the means is always equals to product of the extreme shown as above, in this case,

| 1 (extreme) | : | 10 (mean) | = | 2 (mean) | : | 20 (extreme) |

| 1 (extreme) | x | 20 (extreme) | = | 10 (mean) | x | 2 (mean) |

$$20 = 20$$

The principle of proportion allows you to solve for any unknown 'number' – normally written as 'x' – in a proportion.

For example: -

$$2 : 20 = 4 : x$$

Step 1. Multiply the known numbers (means)

$$20 \times 4 = 80$$

Step 2. Set up the products of the means and extremes in an equation as shown below:-

$$80 = 2x$$

Step 3. Find out the unknown number 'x'

$$\text{Therefore } x = \frac{80}{2} = 40$$

$$x = 40$$

Exercise 10

Find the values of x:

1) $3:6 = 70:x$

2) $4:5 = 44:x$

3) $2:6 = 12:x$

4) $5:3 = 36:x$

5) $3:8 = 54:x$

6) $5:7 = 13:x$

7) $3:4 = 9:x$

8) $4:5 = 70:x$

9) $10:1 = 43:x$

10) $8:3 = 60:x$

The understanding of ratios and proportions are useful in solving the following example problem.

If you were required to dilute liquid A to liquid B in the ratio 1:2 and there was 30 ml of liquid A, then the amount of liquid B required can be worked out using the concepts learned above:

$$1 : 2 = \text{ratio given}$$
$$30 : y = \text{amounts given}$$

y represents the amount of liquid B that is needed.

$$1 : 2 = 30 : y$$
$$2 \times 30 = y \times 1$$
$$60 = y$$

So in the ratio 1:2, you would use 30 ml for liquid A, and 60 ml for liquid B.

A **proportion** can be represented as a fraction, ratio, percentage and decimal.

E.g. $\frac{2}{4}$ (fraction), 2:4 (ratio), 50% (percentage) and 0.5 (decimal) all represent the same proportion.

Exercise 11

Fill in the missing blanks:

	Fraction	Ratio	Percentage	Decimal
1)	$\frac{3}{4}$			
2)		1:2		
3)			37.5%	
4)				0.55
5)	$\frac{6}{8}$			
6)		1:4		
7)			12.5%	
8)				0.4
9)	$\frac{1}{5}$			

Exercise 11 (continued)

Fill in the missing blanks:

	Fraction	Ratio	Percentage	Decimal
10)		2:3		
11)			16%	
12)				0.8
13)	$\frac{9}{10}$			
14)		1:3		
15)			100%	
16)				0.7
17)	$\frac{3}{5}$			
18)		1:10		
19)			45%	
20)				0.01

CHAPTER THREE

> **Learning Outcomes**
>
> At the end of this chapter, you will understand: -
>
> ❖ Converting metric units of weight in respect of prescribed dosages of both oral and non-oral (injections) medications.

The metric system of measurement has been used throughout the hospitals in the United Kingdom since 1975 and yet many nurses are still unsure how to convert from one unit of measurement to another. Incorrect placement of the decimal point can result in errors that are 10 or 100 times the correct dose and mistakes can have fatal consequences for patients.

The gram (g) is the basic metric unit of weight used in pharmaceutical weighing of drugs. The only subdivisions of a gram commonly used are the milligram (mg or 0.001g) and the microgram (mcg or 0.001mg).

The following are some of the very common problems encountered by many nurses. Many nurses are unsure of: -

1) Relative values between these units. (g, mg and mcg)

For example, when asked to convert from milligram (mg) to microgram (mcg), some nurses move the decimal point in the wrong direction because they are not familiar with the metric system.

The following are some of the common mistakes made by some nurses:-

a) 5 g = ? mg

The answers frequently given is 500 mg (Multiply by 100 rather than 1000)

(The correct answer should have been 5 x 1000 = 5000 mg) (Remember 1 g = 1000 mg)

b) 5 mg = ? mcg

The answer frequently given is 500 mcg (Multiply by 100 rather than 1000)

The correct answer should have been 5 x 1000 = 5000 mcg (Remember 1mg = 1000 mcg)

2. Which way they should move the decimal point when converting one unit to another.

The following are some of the common mistakes made by nurses:-

a) 5g = ? mg

The answer frequently given is 0.005 mg (Dividing rather than multiplying by 1000)?

The correct answer should have been 5 x 1000 = 5000 mg (Remember 1 g = 1000 mg therefore we must multiply by 1000, thus moving the decimal point forward)

b) 5mg = ? mcg

The answer frequently given is 0.005 mcg (Dividing rather than multiplying by 1000)

The answer should have been 5 x 1000 = 5000 mcg (Remember 1 mg = 1000 mcg therefore we must multiply by 1000, thus moving the decimal point forward)

3. If they know which way to move the decimal point, they do not know how many decimal places to move it.

For example,

a) 5 g = ? mg

The answer frequently given is 500 mg (The decimal point has only been moved 2 places forward).

The answer should have been 5 x 1000 = 5000 mg (Remember 1g = 1000 mg therefore to show a multiplication by 1000 the decimal point must be moved 3 places forward)

b) 5 mg = ? mcg

The answer frequently given is 500 mcg (The decimal point has been moved only 2 places forward).

The answer should have been 5 x 1000 = 5000 mcg
(Remember 1 mg = 1000 mcg therefore to show a multiplication by 1000 the decimal point must be moved 3 places forward)

c) 5 mg = ? g

The answer frequently given is 0.05 g (The decimal point has only been moved 2 places backward).

The answer should have been 5 ÷ 1000 = 0.005g
(Remember 1 mg = $\frac{1}{1000}$ g (1 ÷ 1000) therefore to show a division by 1000 the decimal point must be moved 3 places backward)

d) 5 mcg = ? mg

The answer frequently given is 0.5 mg (The decimal point has been moved only 1 place backward)

The answer should have been 5 ÷ 1000 = 0.005 mg
(Remember 1 mcg = $\frac{1}{1000}$ mg (1 ÷ 1000) therefore to show a division by 1000 the decimal point must be moved 3 places backward)

Summary

A SIMPLE FORMULA TO MEMORISE FOR EASY CONVERSION OF METRIC UNITS OF WEIGHT: -

a) You must place gram (g)   =   One letter
              milligram (mg)   =   Two letters
              microgram (mcg)   =   Three letters

in a logical sequence as shown by the diagram below: -

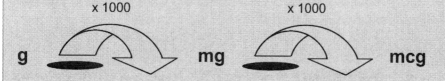

Summary (continued)

b) Therefore, to convert gram to milligram, you simply multiply by 1000 (i.e. move the decimal point three places to the right (forward)).

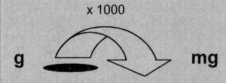

For example, convert 5 g to mg

Therefore, the answer is 5 g = 5 x 1000

= 5.000. mg
= 5000 mg

c) To convert milligram (mg) to microgram (mcg) you also multiply by 1000 (i.e. move the decimal point three places to the right (forward)).

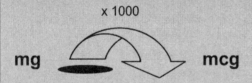

For example, convert 5 mg to mcg

Therefore, the answer is 5 mg = 5 x 1000

= 5.000. mcg
= 5000 mcg

d) However, if you want to convert mg to g, you would have to divide by 1000 (i.e. move the decimal point three places to the left (backward)).

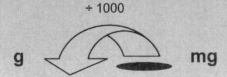

Summary (continued)

For example, convert 5 mg to g

Therefore, the answer is 5 mg = 5 ÷ 1000

= 0.005. g
= 0.005 g

e) Likewise, if you want to convert mcg to mg, you would have to divide by 1000 (i.e. move the decimal point three places to the left (backward)).

÷ 1000

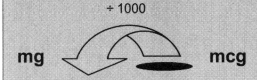

mg   **mcg**

For example, convert 5 mcg to mg

Therefore, the answer is 5 mcg = 5 ÷ 1000

= 0.005. mg
= 0.005 mg

When converting metric units (measurement of weight) the following diagram should be memorised: -

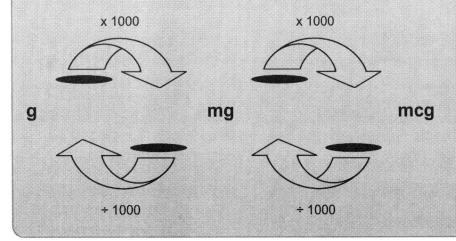

x 1000   x 1000

g   **mg**   **mcg**

÷ 1000   ÷ 1000

Exercise 1

Very often a doctor may prescribe in "milligram" but the stock dose is labelled as "micrograms", therefore, the milligram would be converted to microgram, similarly the prescription may be in "gram" but the stock dose is labelled "milligram", therefore the gram would be converted to milligram.

Correctly convert the following drug dosages.

1) 0.0625 mg of digoxin	=	mcg
2) 500 mcg of digoxin	=	mg
3) 125 mcg of digoxin	=	mg
4) 0.25 mg of digoxin	=	mcg
5) 100 mcg of eltroxin	=	mg
6) 150 mcg of morphine	=	mg
7) 2 mg of morphine	=	mcg
8) 200 mcg of morphine	=	mg
9) 25 mcg of lorazepam	=	mg
10) 4 mg of lorazepam	=	mcg
11) 3 mg of buprenorphine	=	mcg
12) 0.4 mg of carbamazepine	=	mcg
13) 500 mcg of dexamethasone	=	mg
14) 500 mg of hydrocortisone	=	mcg
15) 2.5 g of methionine	=	mg
16) 500 mg of paracetamol	=	g
17) 20 mcg of naloxone	=	mg
18) 1.5 g of benzylpenicillin	=	mg
19) 500 mcg of terbutamide	=	mg
20) 0.01 mg of dobutamine	=	mcg
21) 0.005 mg dopamine	=	mcg
22) 0.6 g of procainamide	=	mg
23) 0.4 g of disopyramide	=	mg
24) 0.05 mg of lanoxin elixir	=	mcg

CHAPTER FOUR

4

> ## Learning Outcomes
>
> At the end of this chapter, you will be able to: -
> * ❖ Convert litres to millilitres and vice versa.

The Litre is the metric volume unit that is frequently used by nurses both on parenteral and non-parenteral drugs. The only subdivision of a Litre commonly used is the millilitre (ml or 0.001 L), in other words 1 L = 1000 ml.

Some nurses are unsure of: -

1. The relative value between (L) and (ml)

For example, when asked to convert from Litre (L) to millilitre (ml), some nurses move the decimal point in the wrong direction because they are not familiar with the metric system.

a) 2.5 L = ? ml

The answer frequently given is 250 ml. (multiplication has been made by 100)

The correct answer should have been 2,500 ml

(Remember - since 1 L = 1000 ml, multiplication must be by 1000, where the decimal point must be moved 3 places forward.)

b) 35 ml = ? L

The answer frequently given is 0.35 L (Division has been made by 100)

The correct answer should have been 0.035 L

(Remember - since 1000 ml = 1 L, division must be by 1000, where the decimal point must be moved 3 places backward.)

2. Which way they should move the decimal point when converting from one unit to another?

For example,

a) 250 ml = ? L

The answer frequently given is 250 L (Obviously no division has taken place - the ml is only $\frac{1}{1000}$ (1 ÷ 1000) L so cannot be equal to it!)

The correct answer should have been 0.25 L

Moving the decimal point 3 places backward shows (Division by 1000.)

b) 2 L = ? ml

The answer frequently given is 0.002 ml (Here division not multiplication has taken place.)

The answer should have been 2000 ml

(If 1 L = 1000 ml then 2 L must be multiplied by 1000 thus moving the decimal point 3 places forward.)

3. Again, even if they know which way they to move the decimal point, they do not know how many decimal places, to move it.

For example,

a) 5 L = ? ml

The answer frequently given is 50 ml (This shows a multiplication of only 10)

The answer should have been 5000 ml

(Since 1 L = 1000 ml then the multiplication must be by 1000, thus moving the decimal point 3 places forward.)

b) 500 ml = ? L

The answer frequently given is 0.05 L (This shows a division of only 10,000)

The answer should have been 0.5 L

(Since 1 ml = $\frac{1}{1000}$ L (1 ÷ 1000), division must be by 1000, thus moving the decimal point 3 places backward.)

Summary

A SIMPLE FORMULA TO MEMORISE FOR EASY CONVERSION OF METRIC UNITS OF FLUID: -

a) You must place Litre (L)   =   One letter

　　　　　　　millilitre (ml)   =   Two letters

In a logical sequence as shown by the diagram below: -

x 1000

L 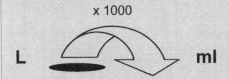 ml

b) Therefore, to convert Litre (L) to millilitre (ml), you simply multiply by 1000 (i.e. move the decimal point three places to the right (forward)).

For example,

3 L = ? ml

3 L = 3 x 1000   = 3.000. ml

　　　　　　　　　= 3000 ml

c) However, if you want to convert millilitre to Litre, you would have to divide by 1000 (i.e. move thedecimal point three places to the left (backward)).

For example,

280 ml = ? L

280 ÷ 1000   = 0.280. L

　　　　　　　　　= 0.28 L

x 1000

L   ml

When converting metric units (weight of fluid) the following should be memorised: -

÷ 1000

Exercise 1

Identify the values of the following:

1) 250 ml = ___ L   8) 23 ml = ___ L   15) 505 ml = ___ L

2) 1.5 L = ___ ml   9) 28.5 ml = ___ L   16) 42.5 ml = ___ L

3) 0.85 L = ___ ml   10) 7.5 ml = ___ L   17) 1.008 L = ___ ml

4) 24.5 ml = ___ L   11) 9.1 ml = ___ L   18) 350 ml = ___ L

5) 2750 ml = ___ L   12) 225 ml = ___ L   19) 0.09 L = ___ ml

6) 750 ml = ___ L   13) 0.15 L = ___ L   20) 2.25 L = ___ ml

7) 0.025 L = ___ ml   14) 0.02 L = ___ ml

CHAPTER FIVE

Accuracy in calculation of drug dosages is essential for the administration of the therapeutic dosage. Inaccurate calculations will result in a dose that is too large or too small. Too much a dose will cause toxic effect and, in extreme cases, death. Too low a dose is ineffective, allowing the illness, or symptom to continue and progress. In either case, the drug is unlikely to have any of the desired effects.

Since drug dosages are not individualised i.e. pre-packed ready for each individual patient, a knowledge of and skill in converting a fraction to a decimal is essential. This is illustrated by the drug formula as shown below: -

Some of the common problems encountered by many nurses are as follows: -

They are unsure of: -

1. How to use the formula.

For example, when nurses are asked to use the drug calculation formula they insert the information in the wrong places as shown below: -

$$\frac{\text{Stock (Available) dose x Dilution (ml)}}{\text{Prescribed dose}}$$

The correct way is: -

$$\frac{\text{Prescribed dose x Dilution (ml)}}{\text{Stock (Available dose)}}$$

Even if you obtain the "right " answer from the calculation, if the available dose and the stock dose are placed in the wrong places in the formula, you will never get the right answer.

2. Even if they know the correct formula they do not know how to apply it i.e. how to multiply a fraction by a whole number.

For example,

a) 35 mg of Pethidine is prescribed, and the stock solution is 100 mg per 2 ml, how much in (ml) should you administer to your patient?

The following are some of the mistakes made by some nurses: -

$$\frac{35}{100} \times 2$$

The answer given is $(35 \times 2) \div (100 \times 2)$

Therefore, you now have $70 \div 200 = 0.35$ ml

(Nurses (and others) frequently multiply both the numerator (the prescribed dose - in this case 35) and the denominator (the stock dose - in this case 100) by the dilution (in this case 2) which would result in administering only half the required amount to the patient.

The correct answer should have been $70 \div 100 = 0.7$ ml

(To multiply a fraction by a whole number, multiply the numerator (35 - the prescribed dose) by the whole number (2 - the dilution) and place the denominator (100 - the stock dose) which remains unchanged.

$$\frac{35}{100} \times 2 = \frac{70}{100} = 0.7 \text{ ml}$$

3. How to simplify a fraction before doing the multiplication.

For example,

a) 625 mg of penicillin is prescribed, and the stock solution is 250 mg per 5 ml, how much in (ml) should you administer to your patient?

The following are some of the mistakes made by some nurses: -

$$\text{Formula} = \frac{\text{Prescribed dose}}{\text{Stock (available dose)}}$$

$$= \frac{625}{250} \times 5$$

$$= (625 \times 5) \div 250$$

$$= 3125 \div 250$$

These big numbers are unmanageable and calculation of these numbers often led to mathematical errors.

$$
\begin{array}{r}
12.5 \\
250\overline{)3125} \\
\underline{250} \\
625 \\
\underline{500} \\
125 \\
\underline{125} \\
0
\end{array}
$$

The correct way to do this is: -

$$
\frac{\overset{125}{\cancel{625}}}{\underset{50}{\cancel{250}}} \times 5
$$

$$
= \frac{\overset{25}{\cancel{125}}}{\underset{10}{\cancel{50}}} \times 5
$$

$$
= \frac{125}{10} = 12.5
$$

$$
= 12.5 \text{ ml}
$$

By reducing these big numbers will lead to a simplified and manageable calculation. Therefore, mathematical errors are avoided.

Exercise 1

1) A patient with heart failure is prescribed with 62.5 mcg of digoxin elixir. The available dose on the ward medicine trolley is 50 mcg per ml. Calculate the correct dosage in ml.

2) A patient is prescribed 175 mg of cytosine arabinoside I.V. The available dose is 100 mg in 5 ml. Calculate the correct dosage in ml.

3) A patient is prescribed 25 mg of Promethazine hydrochloride suspension. The available dose is 6.25 mg in 5 ml. Calculate the correct dosage in ml.

4) A patient is prescribed 40 mg of Frusemide. The available dose is 50 mg in 5ml. Calculate the correct dosage.

Exercise 1 (continued)

5) A patient is prescribed 500 mg of Amoxycillin elixir. The available dose is 250mg in 5 ml. Calculate the correct dosage.

6) A patient is prescribed 0.0625 mg of Digoxin elixir. The available dose is 0.05 mg per ml. Calculate the correct dose.

7) A patient is prescribed 450 mg of soluble aspirin. The available dose is 300 mg per tablet. Calculate the correct dosage.

8) A patient is prescribed I.V. 450 mg of Benzl Penicillin. The available dose is 600 mg in 10ml. Calculate the correct dosage.

9) A patient is prescribed 125 mg of Ampicillin. The available dose is 250 mg in 5 ml. Calculate the correct dosage.

10) A patient is prescribed 450 mg of Aspirin elixir. The available dose is 150 mg in 5 ml. Calculate the correct dosage.

11) A patient is prescribed 15 mg of Morphine Sulphate syrup. The available dose is 10 mg in 5 ml. Calculate the correct dosage.

12) A patient is prescribed 50 mg of Getamicin I.V. The available dose is 80 mg in 2 ml. Calculate the correct dosage.

13) A patient is prescribed 1 mg of Mithramycin. The available dose is 2.5 mg in 5 ml. Calculate the correct dosage.

14) A patient is prescribed 125 mg of Erythromycin. The available dose is 500 mg in 10ml. Calculate the correct dosage.

15) A patient is prescribed 75 mg of Pethidine. The available dose is 100 mg in 2 ml. Calculate the correct dosage.

16) A patient is prescribed 400 mg of Aminophylline I.V. The available dose is 250 mg in 10ml. Calculate the correct dosage.

17) A patient is prescribed 500 mg of Penicillin elixir. The available dose is 250 mg in 5ml. Calculate the correct dosage.

Exercise 1 (continued)

18) A patient is prescribed 1.7 g of Mesna. The available dose is 400 mg in 4 ml. Calculate the correct dosage.

19) A patient is prescribed 40 mg of Methotrexate. The available dose is 50 mg in 2 ml. Calculate the correct dosage.

20) A patient is prescribed 6 mg of Diazepam syrup. The available dose is 2 mg in 5 ml. Calculate the correct dosage.

21) A patient is prescribed 0.5 mg of Adrenaline. The available dose is 1 mg in 10 ml. Calculate the correct dosage.

22) A patient is prescribed 10 mg of Pethidine. The available dose is 50 mg in 1 ml. Calculate the correct dosage.

23) A patient is prescribed 0.4 mg of Buprenorphine. The available dose is 300 mcg in 1 ml. Calculate the correct dosage.

24) A patient is prescribed Diazepam 10 mg. The available dose is 5 mg in 2 ml. Calculate the correct dosage.

25) A patient is prescribed 2 mg of Narcan. The available dose is 400 mcg in 1 ml. Calculate the correct dosage.

26) A patient is prescribed 45 mg of Terfenadine. The available dose is 30 mg in 1 ml. Calculate the correct dosage.

27) A patient is prescribed 75 mg of Amitriptylline Hydrochloride. The available dose is 25 mg in 5 ml. Calculate the correct dosage.

28) A patient is prescribed Anafranil 100 mg. The available dose is 25 mg in 5 ml. Calculate the correct dosage.

29) A patient is prescribed Lopresor 150 mg. The available dose is 50 mg per tablet. Calculate the correct dosage.

30) A patient is prescribed Maxolon 10 mg. The available dose is 5 mg in 5 ml. Calcualte the correct dosage.

Summary

A patient is prescribed 25 mg of Promethazine hydrochloride. The available dosage is 2.5 mg in 1 ml. Calculate the correct dosage in ml.

By using the formula:

$$\frac{\text{Prescribed dose}}{\text{Available dose}} \times \text{Dilution}$$

$$\frac{25}{2.5} \times 1 = \frac{\overset{10}{\cancel{25}}}{\underset{1}{\cancel{2.5}}} \times 1 = 10 \text{ ml}$$

CHAPTER SIX

> **Learning Outcomes**
>
> At the end of this chapter, you will be able to: -
>
> ❖ Understand how to accurately calculate the infusion flow rate for blood and fluids in a variety of intravenous giving sets by using a formula.

Accuracy in calculating intravenous fluids is essential if nurses were to deliver therapeutic fluid level required by a patient. Inaccurate calculations will inevitably result in a flow rate that is either too slow or too fast. In each case, it does the patient no good. Too much fluid mistakenly given can overload a patient's heart and in extreme cases can cause death. On the other hand, too little fluid is ineffective and this can cause dehydration, electrolyte imbalance and confusion.

Flow rates are expressed as volumes of fluid delivered per unit of time, usually as millilitres per hour or drops per minute. What you need to know before calculating the flow rate in any given infusion is: -

❖ The total volume of fluid to be infused.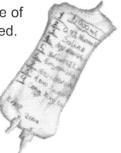

❖ The total infusion time (Hour or Minute).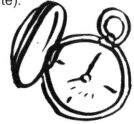

❖ The calibration of the administration set.

For example, 15 drops/ml for blood administration sets.

◆◆◆◆◆
◆◆◆◆◆ = 1ml
◆◆◆◆◆

20 drops/ml for solution administration sets. 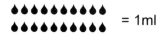 = 1ml

60 mini-drops/ml for burettes and solution administration sets. (The information is found on the administration set package)

♦♦♦♦♦♦♦♦♦♦♦♦♦♦♦
♦♦♦♦♦♦♦♦♦♦♦♦♦♦♦   = 1ml
♦♦♦♦♦♦♦♦♦♦♦♦♦♦♦

Some of the common problems encountered by some nurses are as follow: -

They are unsure of: -

1. How to use the infusion flow rate formula.

For example, when nurses are asked to use the infusion flow rate formula they insert the information in the wrong places as shown below: -

$$\text{Flow rate (drops/min)} = \frac{\text{Total volume of fluid}}{\text{Total infusion time [no. of hours x 60 x calibration (drops/ml)]}}$$

The correct way is: -

$$\text{Flow rate (drops/min)} = \frac{\text{Total volume of fluid x calibration (drops/ml)}}{\text{Total infusion time (no. of hours x 60)}}$$

1. Even if you obtain the 'right' answer from the calculation, if the calibration (drop/ml) is placed in the wrong in the wrong place, you will **never** get the correct answer.

2. Even they know the formula; some nurses do not know how to apply it i.e. how to multiply a fraction by a whole number.

For example, 1000 ml of normal saline is prescribed intravenously to run over a period of 8 hours, how many drops /min should you administer to your patient?

$$\frac{1000 \times 20}{8 \times 60 \times 20}$$

The answer given is (1000 x 20) ÷ (8 x 60 x 20)

Therefore, you now have 20,000 ÷ 9,600 = 2.08 drops/min

The mistake made by some nurses is that they multiply both the numerator - the prescribed total volume of fluid, in this case 1000 and the denominator - (the total infusion time (min), in this case 8 x 60 = 480) by the calibration (drops/ml), in this case 20.

The correct answer should have been (1000 x 20) ÷ (8 x 60) = 41.66... drops/min.

From these examples, we can learn some key very important principles: -

❖ Keep the calculation as simple as possible.

❖ Anything done to the top of a fraction (Numerator) must also be done to the bottom (Denominator).

❖ Divide and multiply small numbers instead of big numbers.

For example,

$$\frac{1000 \times 20}{8 \times 60} = \frac{1000 \times 1}{8 \times 3} = \frac{500 \times 1}{4 \times 3}$$

$$\frac{250 \times 1}{2 \times 3} = \frac{125 \times 1}{1 \times 3} = \frac{125}{3} = 41.66...$$

Since it is difficult to think in terms of drops per min., we can convert 41.66 to ml (there are 20 drops in 1 ml) by dividing 20. (use your calculator)

41.6666 divide 20 = 2.083 ml/min.

Therefore, in one hour's time = 60 x 2.083 = 124.99999

In 8 hours, time = 8 x 124.99999 = 999.9999 = 1000 ml (The original amount)

By using this method, you can check whether your answer is worked out correctly!

Exercise 1

Calculation on infusion flow rate

Calculate the following flow rate in drops/min. The intravenous giving set delivers 20 drops/ml

1) 1000 ml of normal saline is prescribed to a patient over 4 hours.

2) 500 ml of dextrose saline is to be given to a patient over 3 hours.

3) A patient is to have 1000 ml of Hartmann's solution over 10 hours.

Exercise 1 (continued)

4) A patient is to have 500 ml of normal saline over 4 hours.

5) A patient is to receive 1000 ml of dextrose saline over 12 hours.

6) A patient is to receive 500 ml of dextrose saline over 12 hours.

7) A patient is to have 250 ml of normal saline over 3 hours.

8) A patient is to receive 1000 ml of normal saline over 5 hours.

9) A patient is to receive 500 ml of 5% of Dextrose over 5 hours.

10) A patient is to receive 1000 ml of Normal saline 0.9% over 6 hours.

Exercise 2

Calculation on infusion flow rate (blood)

Calculate the following flow rate (drops/min). The intravenous blood administration set delivers 15 drops/ml

1) A patient is to receive 450 ml of blood over 4 hours.

2) A patient with anaemia is to receive 500 ml of blood over 6 hours.

3) A patient is to have 500 ml of blood over 3 hours.

4) A post-operative patient is to receive 500 ml of blood over 5 hours.

5) A patient is to have 250 ml of blood over 3 hours.

6) A patient is to have 350 ml of packed cells over 4 hours.

7) A patient is to receive 450 ml of blood over 6 hours.

8) A patient is to receive 500ml of blood over 4 hours.

9) A patient is to receive 450 ml of blood over 3 hours.

10) A patient is to receive 250 ml of blood over 2 hours.

Exercise 3

Calculation of flow rate on small child

Calculate the following flow rate in (drops/min). The Solution giving set delivers 60 mini-drops/ml

1) A child is to receive 500 ml of Normal Saline 0.9% over 6 hours.

2) A child is to receive 500 ml of Dextrose 5% over 12 hours.

3) A child is to receive 250 ml of Normal Saline 0.9% and Dextrose 0.18% over 4 hours.

4) A child is to receive 300 ml of Dextrose 5% over 6 hours.

5) A child is to receive 600 ml of Normal Saline 0.9% over 8 hours.

6) A child is to receive 400 ml of Dextrose 5% over 5 hours.

7) A child is to receive 200 ml of Normal Saline 0.9% over 5 hours.

8) A child is to receive 500 ml of Dextrose 5% over 9 hours.

9) A child is to receive 350 ml of Normal Saline 0.9% over 5 hours.

10) A child is to receive 450 ml of Dextrose 5% over 5 hours.

When calculating the flow rate in ml per hour, you need to use the following formula.

$$\text{Flow rate (ml per hour)} = \frac{\text{Total volume of fluid}}{\text{Number of hours}}$$

For example, if a patient is to receive 1000 ml of fluid over 4 hours, find out the amount to be given each hour:

$$\text{Flow rate (ml per hour)} = \frac{1000 \text{ ml}}{4 \text{ hours}} = 250 \text{ ml per hour}$$

Exercise 4

Calculating the flow rate (ml per hour)

1) A patient is to receive 1000 ml of Normal saline 0.9% over 10 hour.

2) A patient is to receive 1000 ml of Dextrose 5% Over 8 hours.

3) A patient is to receive 500 ml of Dextrose 4% and Normal saline 0.9% over 4 hours.

4) A patient is to receive Normal saline 1000 ml over 12 hours.

5) A patient is to receive 1000 ml of Normal saline 0.9% over 6 hours.

6) A patient is to receive 1000 ml of Normal saline 0.9% over 5 hours.

7) A patient is to receive 1000 ml of Normal saline 0.9% over 9 hours.

8) A patient is to receive 1000 ml of Dextrose 5% over 11 hours.

9) A patient is to receive 500 ml of Normal saline over 5 hours.

10) A patient is to receive 500 ml of Dextrose 5% over 3 hours.

CHAPTER SEVEN

> **Learning Outcomes**
>
> At the end of this chapter, you will be able to: -
> * Understand how to accurately calculate the flow rate for a drug in an infusion fluid.

Isosorbide Dinitrate solution 0.02% in dextrose saline is to be given to a patient at 0.1 mg/min in a solution administration set with a calibration of 60 drops/ml.

Step 1:   Available dose, Isosorbide dinitrate 0.02 %

          = 0.02 g in 100 ml
          = 20 mg in 100ml

Step 2:   Prescribed doses 0.1 mg/min

Step 3:   Formula = $\dfrac{\text{Prescribed dose}}{\text{Available dose}}$ x Dilution

          $\dfrac{0.1 \text{ mg}}{20}$ x 100 = 0.5 ml

Step 4:   Solution set delivers 60 drops/ml

Therefore flow rate (drops/min) = 0.5 ml x 60 = 30 drops/min.

It is important to understand that when you administer 0.5 ml of this solution, you are giving 0.1 mg of Isosorbide Dinitrate. Similarly, when you administer 30 drops (I.V. set delivers 60 drops/ml), you are also giving 0.1 mg of Isosorbide Dinitrate.

Exercise 1

1) A patient is prescribed Lignocaine 0.4% to be administrered at a rate of 4mg/min. for 30min.

a) Calculate the flow rate in drops/min (In this case, the I.V. set delivers 60 minidrops/ml).
b) Calculate the flow rate in drops/min (In this case, the I.V. set delivers 20 drops/ml).

2) A patient is prescribed Lignocaine 0.4% to be administered at a rate of 2mg/min. for 60 min.

a) Calculate the flow rate in drops/min (In this case, the I.V. set delivers 60 mini-drops/ml.
b) Calculate the flow rate in drops/min (In this case, the I.V. set delivers 20 drops/ml).

3) A patient is prescribed Lidocaine 0.1% to be administered at a rate of 4 mg/min. for 30 min.

a) Calculate the flow rate in drops/min (In this case, the I.V. set delivers 60 mini-drops/ml).
b) Calculate the flow rate in drops/min. (In this case, the I.V. set delivers 20 drops/ml).

4) A patient is prescribed Lidocaine 0.1% to be administered at a rate of 2 mg/min for 2 hours.

a) Calculate the flow rate in drops/min. (In this case, the I.V. set delivers 60 mini-drops/ml).
b) Calculate the flow rate in drops/min. (In this case, the I.V. set delivers 20 mini-drops/ml).

5) A patient is prescribed Lidocaine 0.2% to be administered at a rate of 4 mg/min for 30 min.

a) Calculate the flow rate in drops/min (In this case, the I.V. set delivers 60 mini-drops/ml).
b) Calculate the flow rate in drops/min (In this case, the I.V. set delivers 20 drops/ml).

Exercise 1 (continued)

6) A patient is prescribed I.V. Ketamine to be administered 30 mcg/kg/min. The available dosage is 1 mg in 1 ml and he weighs 40 kg.

a) Calculate the total dosage he will require in 1 min.
b) Calculate the flow rate in drops/min. (In this case, the I.V. set delivers 60 mini-drops/ml).
c) Calculate the flow rate in drops/min. (In this case, the I.V. set delivers 20 drops/ml).

7) A patient is prescribed Diprivan 1% to be administered 0.5 mg/kg/min. and he weighs 60 kg.

a) Calculate the total dosage he will require in 1 min.
b) Calculate the flow rate in drops/min. (In this case, the I.V. set delivers 20 drops/ml).

8) A patient is prescribed I.V. Renifentanil 0.5 mcg/kg/min. and he weighs 80 kg. The available dosage is 1 mg in 1 ml.

a) Calculate the total dosage he will require in 1 min.
b) Calculate the flow rate in drops/min. (In this case, the I.V. set delivers 60 mini-drops/ml).

9) A patient is prescribed I.V. Thiopental Sodium 2.5% to be administered at a rate of 2mg/kg and the patient weighs 50 kg.

a) Calculate the total dosage he will require.
b) Calculate the flow rate in drops/min. (In this case, the I.V. set delivers 60 drops/ml).

10) A patient is prescribed I.V. Dobutamine 10 mcg/kg/min. and he weighs 60 kg. The available dosage is 500 mg in 250 ml.

a) Calculate the total dosage he will require in 1 min.
b) Calculate the flow rate in drops/min (In this case, the I.V.set delivers 60 drops/ml).

Exercise 1 (continued)

11) A patient is prescribed I.V.Aminophylline 1 mg/kg/hour intermittenatly for 30min. This patient weighs 50 kg.

a) Calculate the total dosage per hour if the available dosage of this drug is 500 mg in 100 ml
b) Calculate the total volume (in ml) you should administer.

12) A patient is prescribed I.V. Aminophylline 0.5 mg/kg/hour continuously for 2 hours. This patient weighs 50 kg.

a) Calculate the total dosage per hour if the available dosage of this drug is 500 mg in 250 ml.
b) Calculate the total volume (in ml) you should administer.

13) A patient is prescribed I.V. Disopyramide 400mcg/kg/hour and he weighs 60 kg.

a) Calculate the total dosage he will need per hour if the available dosage is 10 mg in 1 ml.
b) Calculate the total volume (in ml) you should administer.

14) A patient is prescribed I.V. Maxolon 2.5mg/kg/hour and he weighs 50 kg.

a) Calculate the total dosage he will per hour if the available dosage is 5mg in 1 ml.
b) Calculate the total volume (in ml) you should administer.

15) A patient is prescribed I.V. Procainamide 30 mg/min. and he weighs 50 kg.

a) Calculate the total dosage he will need per hour if the available dosage is 100 mg in 1 ml.
b) Calculate the total volume (in ml) you should administer.

Exercise 1 (continued)

16) A patient is prescribed I.V. Diazoxide 2 mg/kg/min for 15 min. and he weighs 30 kg.

   a) Calculate the total dosage he will need if the available dosage is 15 mg in 1 ml.
   b) Calculate the total volume (in ml) you should administer.

17) A patient is prescribed I.V. Lorazepam 50 mcg/kg for the first 30 min. and he weighs 60 kg.

   a) Calculate the total dosage he will need if the available dosage is 4 mg in 1 ml.
   b) Calculate the total volume (in ml) you should administer.

18) A patient is prescribed I.V. Mivacurium 100 mcg/kg for 15 min. and he weighs 50 kg.

   a) Calculate the total dosage he will need if the available dosage is 2 mg in 1 ml.

19) A patient is prescribed I.V. Suxamethonium Chloride 1 mg/kg and he weighs 50 kg.

   a) Calculate the total dosage he will need if the available dosage is 2 mg in 1 ml.
   b) Calculate the total volume (in ml) you should administer.

20) A patient Esmolo Hydrochloride 150 mcg/kg/min. and he weighs 60 kg.

   a) Calculate the total dosage he will need if the available dosage is 10mg in 1 ml.
   b) Calculate the total dosage (in ml) you should administer.

CHAPTER EIGHT

8

RATIOS AND PERCENTAGES

> **Learning Outcomes**
>
> At the end of this chapter, you will be able to: -
>
> ❖ Understand how to accurately convert the ratios and percentages of drugs.

Ratios

Some drugs are labelled as ratios. The ratio of a drug is its dilution strength. For example, adrenaline has two standard strengths: 1-ml ampoule of 1 in 1000 and 10 ml ampoule of 1 in 10,000. Ratio may also be written with colons like 1: 1000 The first number represents the weight in gram; the second represents the volume in millilitres.

So, 1 in 1000 adrenaline means that there is 1 gram of adrenaline in every 1000 ml of solution. This can rewritten as $\frac{1g}{1000ml}$ or 1000 mg in 1000 ml; so $\frac{1000mg}{1000ml} = \frac{1}{1}$. or 1 mg per ml. The ampoule contains 1ml, so there is 1 mg of Adrenaline in the ampoule.

Exercise 1

Find out how many milligrams in 1 millilitre:

1) Adrenaline 1 in 200,000

2) Adrenaline 1 in 80,000

3) Chlorhexidine 1 in 5000

4) Hibicet 1 in 100

5) Disodium Edetate 1 in 10,000

6) Medication of a drug is 1 in 20,000

Exercise 1 (continued)

7) Medication of a drug is 1 in 50,000

8) Medication of a drug is 1 in 8,000

9) Medication of a drug is 1 in 4,000

10) Medication of a drug is 1 in 60,000

Exercise 2

Find out the amount of drug in mg in the volume specified for the following solutions:-

1) 10 ml of a 10% solution	11) 50 ml of 2.5% solution
2) 20 ml of a 0.2% solution	12) 125 ml of 2% solution
3) 5 ml of a 20% solution	13) 60 ml of 5 % solution
4) 100 ml of a 0.1% solution	14) 100 ml of 0.38% solution
5) 100 ml of a 0.9% solution	15) 100 ml of 2.8 % solution
6) 1000 ml of a 0.18 % solution	16) 10 ml of 25% solution
7) 500 ml of 0.5 % solution	17) 60 ml of 0.75 % solution
8) 40 ml of 10% solution	18) 200 ml of 0.5% solution
9) 100 ml of 1% solution	19) 300 ml of 0.5 % solution
10) 100 ml of 0.01% solution	20) 200 ml of 3% solution

Percentage concentration (drug concentration) Some drugs are expressed or labelled as percentages (%). This represents weight in volume in grams per 100 ml of solution. This is independent of the size of the container. So, 0.9 % of normal saline has 0.9 gram of sodium chloride dissolved in every 100 ml of fluid. This will remain the same regardless of if it is in a 10 ml ampoule, 500 ml or 1 litre infusion bag.

Exercise 3

Calculate the amount of electrolyte content or drug (in g and mg) in the volumes specified in the following: -

1) 5% Glucose

2) 0.45% Sodium Chloride

3) 0.225% Sodium Chloride

4) 0.18% Sodium Chloride

5) 4% Glucose

6) 10% Glucose

7) 2.5% Mannitol

8) Dextran 6%

9) 3.86% Glucose

10) Chlorhexidine Mouth wash 0.2%

11) Hexetidine Mouth wash 0.1%

12) Benzydamide oral rinse 0.15%

13) Prednisolone eye drops 0.05%

14) Phenylmercuric nitrate 0.001%

15) Bupivacaine Hydrochloride 0.375%

16) Hydroxyethlcellulose 0.44%

17) Isopto Frin 0.12%

18) Zacin 0.025%

19) Capsicum Oleoresin 0.035%

20) Potassium Chloride 0.0075%

Example: -

Express 100 mg in 1 ml

Since all solution is in 100 ml solution you need to multiply 1 ml by 100. You need to multiply 100 mg by 100 as well. Therefore, there are 100 mg x 100 in 1ml x 100 = 10,000 mg in 100 ml.

$$= \frac{10,000}{1000} = 10 \text{ g} = \textbf{10\%}$$

You can do this by using ratio:-

100 mg = 1 ml

100 mg x 100 = 1 ml x 100

10,000 mg = 100 ml

$\frac{10,000 \text{ mg}}{1000}$ = 10 g in 100 ml = **10%**

Exercise 4

Express the following solute in a solution in percentage: -

1) 2 g in 10 ml	=	%	11) 5 mg in 5ml	=	%
2) 2.5 g in 50 ml	=	%	12) 50 mg in 5 ml	=	%
3) 3 g in 10 ml	=	%	13) 500 mcg in 1 ml	=	%
4) 200 mg in 1 ml	=	%	14) 4 mg in 1 ml	=	%
5) 100 mg in 100 ml	=	%	15) 50 mcg in 1 ml	=	%
6) 15 g in 1000 ml	=	%	16) 250 mg in 5 ml	=	%
7) 20 mg in 1 ml	=	%	17) 24 mg in 1 ml	=	%
8) 1.5 g in 15 ml	=	%	18) 500 mg in 5 ml	=	%
9) 10 mg in 5 ml	=	%	19) 40 mg in 5 ml	=	%
10) 125 mg in 5 ml	=	%	18) 50 mg in 1 ml	=	%

CHAPTER NINE

9

PAEDIATRIC DOSAGE

> **Learning Outcomes**
>
> At the end of this chapter, you will be able to: -
>
> ❖ Understand how to accurately calculate the drug dosages for children.

Great care must be taken especially when administering drugs for young children as their range of weights is so wide. As compared to an adult, the dosage of many drugs is much smaller than the dosage of same drug for an adult.

Children's drug doses are more often prescribed in relation to body weight. The most accurate of calculating a child's dose is to base on his/her body weight in kilogram multiply by the recommended dose of a drug. In most cases the dose is prescribed on a 24 - hour period of time and then divided into an equal number of doses.

For example: A child weighs 44 lb. is prescribed the recommended dose of Penicillin V 50mg/kg/day and is to be given 4 times a day. Find out the correct dose for a single dose.

You need to find out the following: -

1) The child's weight in kilogram.
   44lb ÷ 2.2 = 20kilogram

2) Multiply the child's weight in kilogram by the recommended dose.
   20 x 50 = 1000 mg/day

3) Then divide the total daily dose by the number of doses for the day.
   1000 ÷ 4 = 250 mg (4 times a day)

Exercise 1

1) A child is prescribed the recommended dose of Ampicillin 80mg/kg/day, 4 doses per day. He weighs 22 lbs.

a) Calculate the total dosage he will require per day.
b) Calculate the size of a single dose.

2) A child is prescribed the recommended dose of Erythromycin 40mg/kg/day, 4 doses day. He weighs 44 lbs.

a) Calculate the total dosage he will require per day.
b) Calculate the size of a single dose.

3) A child is prescribed the recommended dose of Gentamycin 3mg/kgdaily, 3 doses per day. He weighs 33 lb.

a) Calculate the total dosage he will require per day.
b) Calculate the size of a single dose.

4) A child with a severe infection is prescribed the recommended dose of Cephradine 75 mg/kg/day, 4 doses per day. He weighs 22 lb.

a) Calculate the total dosage he will require per day.
b) Calculate the size of a single dose.

5) A child with anaemia is prescribed the recommended dose of Folic Acid 500 mcg/kg/daily. He weighs 22 lbs.

a) Calculate the total dosage he will require per day.

6) A child with allergic rhinitis is prescribed the recommended dose of Terfernadine 1 mg/kg/day, 2 doses per day. He weighs 33 lbs.

a) Calculate the total dosage he will require per day.
b) Calculate the size of a single dose.

Exercise 1 (continued)

7) A child with epilepsy is prescribed the recommended dose of Valproate 25 mg/kg/daily, 2 doses per day. He weighs 22 lbs.

a) Calculate the total dosage he will require per day.
b) Calculate the size of a single dose.

8) A child with a gastric condition is prescribed the recommended dose of Dyspamet 20 mg/kg/daily, 3 doses per day. He weighs 33 lbs.

a) Calculate the total dosage he will require per day.
b) Calculate the size of a single dose.

9) A child is prescribed the recommended dose of 50 mg/kg/daily, 4 doses per day. He weighs 17.6 lbs.

a) Calculate the total dosage he will require per day.
b) Calculate the size of a single dose.

10) A child is prescribed the recommended dose of Cefixime 8mg/kg/day, 2 doses per day. He weighs 11 lbs.

a) Calculate the total dosage he will require per day.
b) Calculate the size of a single dose.

Exercise 2

1) A child with a knee infection is prescribed with 75 mg of Flucloxacillin orally. The stock solution is 125 mg of Flucloxacillin in 5 ml. Calculate the correct dose.

2) A child with a cardiac condition prescribed with 30 mcg of Digoxin elixir. The stock solution is 50 mcg of Digoxin in 1 ml. Calculate the correct dose.

Exercise 2 (continued)

3) A child with epilepsy is prescribed with 48 mg of Phenytoin elixir. The stock solution is 30 mg of Phenytoin in 5 ml. Calculate the correct dose.

4) A child with a throat infection is prescribed with I.V. 100 mg of Benzylpenicillin. The stock solution is 600 mg of Benzylpenicillin in 5 ml. Calculate the correct dose.

5) A child is prescribed 80 mg of Paracetamol elixir for his pyrexial. The stock solution is 100 mg of Paracetamol is 5 ml. Calculate the correct dose.

6) A child is prescribed Pethidine 35 mg I.M. for his pain. The stock solution is 50 mg of pethidine in 1 ml. Calculate the correct dose.

7) A child is prescribed 40 mcg of Digoxin. The stock solution is 50 mcg of Digoxin in 2 ml. Calculate the correct dose.

8) A child is prescribed 125 mg of Streptomycin I.M. The stock solution is 1 g of Streptomycin in 2 ml. Calculate the correct dose.

9) A child is prescribed with Penicillin 300 mg. The stock solution is 125 mg of Penicillin in 5 ml. Calculate the correct dose.

10) A child is prescribed Clindamycin 75 mg. The stock solution is 125 mg of Clindamycin in 1ml. Calculate the correct dose.

11) A child with vitamin deficiency is prescribed Folic Acid 500 mcg. The stock is 250 mcg per tablet. Calculate the correct dosage.

12) A child with hay fever is prescribed Terfenadine 0.8 mg. The stock solution is 500 mcg in 5 ml. Calculate the correct dosage.

13) A child with juvenile arthritis is prescribed Ibuprofen 300 mg. The stock solution is 100 mg in 5 ml. Calculate the correct dosage.

14) A child diagnosed with nocturnal enuresis is prescribed Oxybutynin Hydrochloride 3 mg. The stock solution is 2.5 mg in 5 ml.

Exercise 2 (continued)

15) A child with asthma is prescribed with 30 mg of Nuelin. The stock solution is 60 mg in 5 ml. Calculate the correct dosage.

16) A child has a pyrexia and he is prescribed with 0.3 g of Paracetamol. The stock solution is 120 mg in 5 ml. Calculate the correct dosage.

17) A child in respiratory distress is prescribed with 100 mcg of narcan. The stock solution is 400 mcg in 1 ml. Calculate the correct dosage.

18) A child with oedema is prescribed with 30 mg of Furosemide. The stock solution is 4 mg in 1 ml. Calculate the correct dosage.

19) A child with a respiratory problem is prescribed with Alupent 15 mg. The stock solution is 10 mg in 5 ml. Calculate the correct dosage.

20) A child with an allergy is prescribed Phenergan 20 mg. The stock solution is 5 mg in 1 ml. Calculate the correct dosage.

CHAPTER TEN

10

Learning Outcomes

At the end of this chapter, you will be able to: -

❖ Understand how to use a syringe driver.

❖ Understand understand how to calculate the correct dosages when using a syringe driver to administer drugs.

A syringe driver is a lightweight, portable, battery-operated device that delivers precise doses of medication mechanically over a set period of time, most commonly 24 hours.

Because of its versatility, the syringe driver has now found a firm footage, in particular, in the palliative setting. It is used to administer continuous subcutaneous infusions of analgesics, either as single medications, or in combination with other medications such as antiemetics, sedatives, or anticholinergics. The syringe driver can also be used in the medical or surgical setting to administer medications like anticoagulants, insulin and bronchodilators.

Currently, there are two Graseby syringe drivers being used throughout the hospitals in the United Kingdom vis-à-vis the MS26 (green panel) and MS16A (blue panel).

The principal difference between the two above syringe drivers is that the MS26 delivers medication at a rate set in mm per 24 hours, whereas the MS16A delivers medication at a rate set in mm per hour. (please note that delivery is based on the length of the liquid and not the volume – this applies to both devices).

Apart from being light, portable and its ability to deliver precise medications, the syringe driver also has other advantages such as: -

❖ Patient's independence
❖ Is comfortable for ambulant patients
❖ Provides a constant plasma concentrations of medications that are necessary to control and manage symptoms
❖ Avoid repeated injections particularly for the very frail and cachetic patients
❖ Aversion to injections
❖ Sustained continuous infusion over 24 hours or even longer

The syringe driver may be used for the following patients with:

- ❖ Persistent nausea or vomiting
- ❖ Oral or pharyngeal lesions
- ❖ Dysphasia
- ❖ Gastro-intestinal mal-absorption
- ❖ Gastro-intestinal obstructions
- ❖ Frailty and cachexia
- ❖ Unconsciousness
- ❖ Patient's autonomy

Setting up a syringe driver for subcutaneous infusion

It is important to spend time to explain to both the patient and his carers with regard to the nature and intention of the procedure prior to commencing a subcutaneous infusion with a syringe driver. The main reason for this is to eliminate any problems and ensure that everyone is fully informed.

Equipment that should be assembled prior to setting up a syringe driver are: a 9V PP3 alkaline long-life battery or Duracell type MN1604; a Luer-lock 10 or 20 ml syringe; an intravenous giving set; an intravenous cannula (23 or 25 G butterfly needle); transparent adhesion dressing like Opsite or Tagaderm); water for injection and a syringe driver.

The common sites for subcutaneous infusions are: the upper chest; outer upper arm; anterior abdomen; and thighs.

Prepare the syringe driver for action

- ❖ Insert a suitable battery as indicated as above
- ❖ Draw up the prescribed medication to a suitable length that is divisible by 24 hours
- ❖ When setting up a syringe driver, always makes sure that there is 50 mm of diluent (water for injection with prescribed medication) before priming the infusion set. Since priming will take up about 2mm of this total, it will leave 48 mm of fluid to be transfused over 24 hours. For infusions that do not require a priming volume, the length should be set at 48
- ❖ Connect the syringe to an intravenous giving set and use an intravenous cannula for injection, as recommended by the manufacturer as stated above – butterfly cannula
- ❖ Set the rate by using the scale on the syringe driver by measuring the distance in mm that the plunger will move.

Calculation of rate setting for a syringe driver

$$\textbf{Set Rate} \quad = \quad \frac{\textbf{Fluid length in mm}}{\textbf{Infusion time in hours}}$$

For example: diamorphine 50 mg is prescribed to a patient to be infused over 24 hours

Step 1.   dissolve diamorphine in sterile water

Step 2.   draw the dissolved diamorphine into a syringe

Step 3.   draw more sterile water into the syringe so that the length in mm is divisible by 24

$$\frac{\text{Total volume of diamorphine (50 mg) dissolved in sterile water} = 48 \text{ mm stroke length}}{\text{Total number of hours} = 24} = 2 \text{ mm/hr}$$

The idea is that the patient will receive an equal fraction of the total dosage of 50 mg of diamorphine each hour. Thus he will not have the total 50 mg of diamorphine until the 24th hour.

CHAPTER ELEVEN

11

The Law, Documentation and Responsibility of nurse regarding drugs

The Law regarding the Misuse of Drugs Act 1971

This act provides the basis of control for certain drugs (Controlled Drugs) because their misuse can give rise to social problems. The regulations give power to certain individuals to possess, produce, supply, prescribe or administer Controlled Drugs in the practice of their professions. They also apply to the selective control (in terms of record keeping, prescription and destruction) to groups of drugs defined in the Schedules. The penalties as applied to offences involving the different drugs are graded according to the harmfulness attributed to a drug when it is misused. Thus, the drugs are defined in the following three classes:

Class A includes: alfentanil, cocaine, dextromoramide, diamorphine, dipipanone, lysergide (LSD), methadone, methylenedixioxymethamfetamine (MDMA), ecstasy), morphine, opium, pethidine, phencyclidine, and class B substances when prepared for injection.

Class B includes: oral amphetamines, barbiturates, codeine, ethylmorphine, glutethimide, pentazocine, phemetrazine and pholcodine.

Class C includes: certain drugs related to the amphetamines such as benfetamine and chlorphetermine, buprenorphine, cannabis, cannabis resin, diethylpropion, mazindol, meprobamate, pemoline, pipradol, most benzodiazepines, androgenic and anabolic steroids, clenbutrol, chorionic gonadotrophin (HCG), non-human chorionic gonadotrophin, somatotropin, somatrem and somatropin.

Class	Description	Examples
Schedule 1	Virtually all the drugs in this group are prohibited, except in accordance with the Home Office authority. All of these have a very high potential for misuse and they are not used medicinally.	Marijuana (Cannabis) and LSD
Schedule 2	Like Schedule 1 drugs, these also have a very high potential for misuse and they can lead to not only the physical but also psychological dependence.	Amphetamine, Cocaine, Diamorphine (Heroin), Morphine and Pethidine.
Schedule 3	Drugs in this group have an even more powerful potential for misuse than Schedule 1 and 2 drugs. As a consequence, they are subject to special prescription requirements.Prescriptions for this group may be repeated if authorised.	Barbiturates, Meprobamate and Pentazocine and Temazepam.
Schedule 4	Drugs in this group have a potential for misuse but at a lower risk than those in Schedule 1 to 3 and they are only subject to a minimum control. These are not subjected to special prescription requirements as in Schedule 3.	Benzodiazepines
Schedule 5	Schedule 5 drugs have a low potential for misuse because of their strengths. For most part, these are preparations that contain a small amount of narcotics so they are exempt from control drug requirements.	Kaolin and Morphine, Codeine Linctus and DF 118 tablets.

The legal controls are:

1. There should be strict entries of receipts and supply with running balance at all times in a pharmacy department.

2. The pharmacy department can only supply to wards on a signed requisition from the nurse-in-charge (must be a 1st level registered nurse). This must specify the total quantity. The pharmacy department and the ward must retain a copy for two years.

3. Drugs can only be administered to a patient by a medical doctor or dentist via a prescription.

4. The controlled drugs must be kept in a locked cupboard within a locked cupboard at all times; the keys to which are held by the nurse-in-charge or pharmacist.

5. All prescriptions for outpatient or discharge must comply with the following: -

    ❖ All writing must be in ink with the doctor's own handwriting
    ❖ Names, address, date and signature
    ❖ The doctor must write clearly the name of the medication to be administered, the dose and the total quantity in words and figures.

6. The destruction of any drugs must be in the presence of an authorised person.

Medicines Act 1968

The Medicines Act 1968 regulates manufacture, sale and supply of all substances, which are used as medicinal products or ingredients in medicinal products. Standards of manufacture are strictly controlled and the quality of all substances and labelling strictly defined.

Classification of Medicinal products in the United Kingdom

General Sales List medicines (GSL)

These need neither a prescription nor the supervision of a pharmacist and can be obtained from retail outlets like Asda and Morrison supermarket e.g. Paracetamol and Antacids.

Pharmacy-Only medicines (P)

Medications that are being sold in pharmacies – A Registered pharmacist must be on duty on the premise at the time of the sale.
E.g. certain compound analgesics and antifungal agents

Prescription-only Medicines (POMs)

Medications are only dispensed to a patient on the instruction of a medical doctor or dentist or from an approved list for a nurse prescriber. When in doubt, the pharmacist is the expert on all aspects of medicines legislation and should be consulted.

Controlled Drugs (CD)

Controlled drugs are under the regulations of Misuse of Drugs Act 1971.

In hospitals, all classes of drugs are prescribed and they are kept locked (Controlled Drugs are being kept separately in a locked cupboard within a locked cupboard) with the exception of nurse prescribed items locally agreed. The registered nurse-in-charge of a ward has the overall accountability for the safekeeping and storage of all medicines in cupboards, trolleys and cabinets.

Ward Drug Storage

1. Internal – Solid dose form like tablets/caplets/capsule
2. Internal – liquids dose like elixir
3. External – liquids applications like
4. Antiseptics and disinfectants
5. Urine testing strips
6. Intravenous (IV) Infusions
7. Cool storage cabinet (separate for IV feeds)
8. Injections – like vials, ampoules and mini-jets

The role of the nurse in administering medications

The UKCC Document Standards for the Administration of Medicines (NMC, 2007) clearly sets out the responsibilities of nurses when they are involved in the administration of medications. However, nurses must also be made aware of their local policies and procedures so that they can administer medications safely.

When administering medications to a patient a nurse must follow the 5 'Rights':-

1. Check that the Right drug is administered (check the name of the drug)

2. To the Right patient (Patient's name, date of birth and hospital number)

3. In the Right dose (must have knowledge of drug calculation formula to calculate the correct dose because not every patient is prescribed with the same dosage as the available stock dose)

4. By the Right route

   ❖ Orally (solid or liquid)
   ❖ Injections - I.V., I.M. S/C or Intradermal
   ❖ Rectally – suppositories, enemas, foams, ointments
   ❖ Inhalations – inhalers and nebulisers
   ❖ Sublingually – GTN
   ❖ Locally – Ointments, creams, pastes, patches

5. At the Right time (Check the right date and time of administration)

According to the UKCC Document for the Administration of Medicines (NMC, 2002) the administration of medicines is not solely a mechanistic task. It involves the cognitive process i.e. a registered nurse must be knowledgeable about the drug that she is administrating. For example, she also needs to know its effects and side-effects, contra-indications and treatments. A registered nurse should know when a drug has achieved its therapeutic effect and it is her responsibility to contact the prescriber to stop the medication. For instance, it is no good carrying on administering frusemide to a patient to treat his gross oedema when in fact he is showing signs of dehydration, disorientation, low blood pressure and depletion of potassium. In other words, the frusemide has done its job to rid the oedema. By carrying on administering frusemide just because it is on the prescription will compromise this patient's health. However, the registered nurse may request the presciber to prescribe a milder diuretic as a maintenance dose to keep the patient's oedema at bay.

CHAPTER TWELVE

> ## Learning Outcomes
>
> At the end of this chapter, you will be able to: -
> * ❖ Understand why tablets should not be crushed and capsules should not be opened.
> * ❖ Avoid common confusions of medications with very similar names.

It is common practice for nurses to crush tablets or open capsules when they find that their patients cannot swallow their tablets or capsules for one reason or another. The reasons for their inability to swallow are: stroke, oesophageal tumours or the stricture of the cardiac sphincter, mouth ulcers or dental problems, confusion or dementia where the patients spit the medications out, and patients on Percutanoeus Endoscopic Gastrostomy (PEG) or NasoGastric (NG) feeds.

However, this practice is no longer acceptable because it is against the law. By crushing the tablets or opening the capsules the physical form of these medications are changed. So what are the dangers? When some capsules are opened they are released into the blood circulation in a much quicker time (e.g. 20 minutes instead of the normal time of 12 hours). As a consequence, the medications become toxic rather than therapeutic. Secondly, it is a health hazard to undertake such a practice. For example, when antibiotic capsules are opened the powder is released in the air and the administrating nurse or any other patient or relative in close proximity can inhale this. This can lead to antibiotic resistance. In addition, the administrating nurse or other patient and relative in immediate vicinity may suffer from allergies due to the powder released from the capsule. For example, when a Tamoxifen tablet is crushed, the powder is released and its hormonal effect can be toxic to the skin. Similarly, it can also cause unnecessary skin allergies. Also, a nurse would normally use two dessert spoons to help crush the tablet. As a result of this, a certain amount of tablet is coated onto the spoons. This means that there is less dose left for the patient. Again, a therapeutic dose is not administered. Finally if spoons, which are used to administer crushed tablets for two patients, are not cleaned between administrations, then there may be a chance of mixing the medications. This will lead to incorrect medication being administered to the second patient.

Some of the medications that should never be crushed or opened are:

1. Modified release, normally identified by two letters m/r (modified release), LA (long acting), SA (short acting), CR, XL or SR (slow release) are medications designed to be released over a long period of time. (Examples are Verapamil, Propanolol, Nifedepine (Adalat retard), Felodipine m/r and Tramadol (Zydol SR) and m/r Dypyridamole.

2. Enteric coated, normally identified by two letters EN or EC (enteric coated) are medications designed not to be released in the stomach as they can cause harm to it. (Examples of these are Diclfenac (Volarol EC), Aspirin (NU-seals), Naproxen (Naprosyn EC) and Sulphasalazine (Salazopyrin EN).

3. Hormonal, cytotoxic and steroidal can be released into the air by crushing and inadvertently received by the administrating nurse. (Examples of these are Tamoxifen (hormone), Methotrexate (cytotoxic) and dexamethasone (steroid).

4. Nitrate can cause potential explosion. (Examples of these are Glyceryl trinitrate (GTN), Isosorbibe mononitrate and Isosorbide dinitrate.

When a tablet does not appear in the BNF (British National Formulary) in a liquid or elixir form it does not mean that the pharmacy does not keep it. Always consult the pharmacist for advice. The principal practice is to ensure patient safety so crushing tablets or opening capsules are not options!

It must be borne in mind that a liquid dose is not always equivalent to the solid dose form. For example, a Phynetoin tablet of 100mg is equivalent to 90 mg of Phynetoin liquid.

There is always the possibility of errors because names of some medications have very similar sounding names. The consequence of administrating a wrong drug can cause unnecessary complications or even death. Listed below are some examples of common confusions but it is far from exhaustive.

❖ Quinidine Sulphate (for treating ventricular arrhythmias) and Quinine Sulphate (for treating malaria and nocturnal leg cramp).

❖ Disopyramide (for treating ventricular arrhythmias) and Dipyridamole (as a adjunct to oral anticoagulant for prophylaxis of thromboembolism associated with prosthetic heart vavles).

- ❖ De-Nol (for treating gastric and duodenal ulcers) and Danol (inhibits pituitary gonadotrophins) or Daonil (an oral antidiabetic drug) or Danazol (inhibits pituitary gonadotrophins).

- ❖ Dopamine (for treating cardiogenic shock) and Dobutamine (inotropic sympathomimetics) or Doxapram (is a central and respiratory stimulant).

- ❖ Chlorpropamide (for treating diabetes mellitus) and Chlorpromazine (antipsychotic).

- ❖ Co-amilozide (diuretic with amiloride and hydrochlorothiazide) and Co-amilofruse (amiloride with furosemide).

- ❖ Promazine (antipsychotic) and Promethazine (nausea, vertigo and motion sickness).

- ❖ Nifedipine (Calcium-channel blocker) and Nimodipine (prevention and treatment of ischaemic neurological deficits following sub-arachnoid haemorrhage) or Nicardipine (prophylaxis of angina and mild to moderate hypertension).

- ❖ Ismo (for angina) and Istin (hypertension and prophylaxis of angina).

CHAPTER THIRTEEN

What are descriptive statistics?

It is important that the results of a study should be given in a form which makes them easily understood by the reader. This can be achieved by creations of comprehensible tables of results or graphical method by a histogram. A second approach of presenting the results to the reader in order that they can be readily comprehensible in relation to descriptive statistics is to summarise certain aspects of the results. There are two types of descriptive statistics that are normally used: ones that give a measure of central tendency – the most typical value and ones that give a measure of dispersion – the variability or spread for a set of results.

Measures of central tendency

The arithmetic mean

The arithmetic mean is the most frequently used measure of the most typical value. It is the average of a set of scores, obtained by adding together all scores and dividing by the number of scores. This can be represented by the use of symbols. For example the scores are normally represented by the symbol 'x'. So the first score is written as x_1, the second is written as x_2....... The total number of scores is written as 'n'. The mean score is written as x, usually referred to as '$\bar{x}$' (x bar).

$$\bar{x} = \frac{\text{Total of all scores}}{\text{Total number of scores}}$$

This can also be expressed as

$$\bar{x} = \frac{\varepsilon x}{n}$$

Where εx means the total of all the x scores.

For example, if the scores are as shown below we can work out the mean, median and mode:

Student	Liz	John	Sam	Ann	Beck	Sal	Luke	Dan	Mark	Lisa
Test Score %	65	40	50	100	95	80	50	50	100	70

Mean	Median	Mode
70	67.5	50

To work out the mean;

$$\bar{x} = \frac{\text{Total of all scores}}{\text{Total number of scores}}$$

Therefore:

$$\bar{x} = \frac{65+40+50+100+95+80+50+50+100+70}{10} = \frac{700}{10} = 70 \qquad \text{The } \textbf{mean} \text{ is } 70$$

The median

The median is a value selected so that it has as many scores above it as it has below it. To find out the median, the scores should be placed in order of size. If the total number of scores is odd, then the median is the central value for example if there are 23 scores it is the twelfth score from either end. However, if the number of scores is even, then the median is normally taken as the arithmetic mean of the two central values.

To work out the median;

The first thing to do is to put the scores in order lowest to highest;

Student	John	Sam	Luke	Dan	Sal	Beck	Ann	Mark
Test Score %	40	50	50	50	80	95	100	100

The total number of scores is 10. This is an even number and so the median is the mean of the two central values.

The two central values are;

Liz   Lisa
65   70

The mean of these two central values is the median which is;

$$\overline{x} = \frac{65 + 70}{2} = 67.5 \qquad \text{The \textbf{median} is \textbf{67.5}}$$

The mode

The mode represents the value that is most frequently occurring in a set of scores. If a histogram is plotted, then the peak of the histogram gives the modal value.

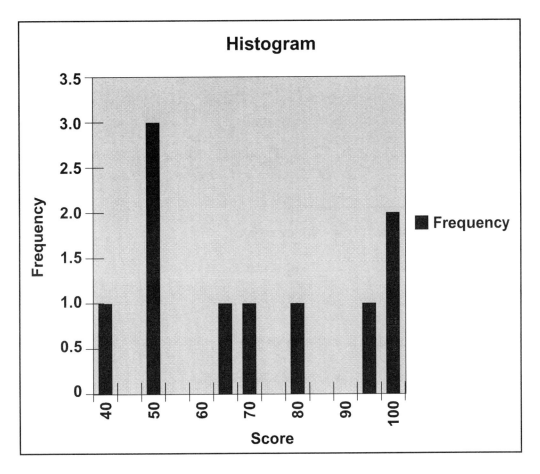

The peak is at 50 so the **mode** for this data is **50**.

Summary - mean, median and mode

The mean is the average of a set of data, obtained by adding together all scores and dividing by the number of data.

The median is the middle number of a set of data.

The mode is the most frequently occurring number of a set of data.

Reference Section

CHAPTER 1

milligram to gram	=	mg ÷ 1000
gram to kilogram	=	g ÷ 1000
gram to milligram	=	g x 1000
kilogram to gram	=	kg x 1000
millilitre to litre	=	ml ÷ 1000
litre to millilitre	=	l x 1000
millimetre to centimetre	=	mm ÷ 10
centimetre to metre	=	cm ÷ 100
metre to kilometre	=	m ÷ 1000
centimetre to millimetre	=	cm x 10
metre to centimetre	=	m x 100
kilometre to metre	=	km x 1000
pounds to kilograms	=	lb ÷ 2.2
kilograms to pounds	=	kg x 2.2

CHAPTER 2

Multiply by 10
When we multiply by 10, we move the decimal point 1 place to the **right.** This makes the number 10 times bigger.

Multiply by 100
When we multiply by 100, we move the decimal point by 2 places to the **right.** This makes the number 100 times bigger.

Multiply by 1000
When we multiply by 1000, we move the decimal point 3 places to the **right.** This makes the number 1000 times bigger.

Divide by 10
When we divide by 10, we move the decimal point 1 place to the **left.** This makes the number smaller 10 times smaller.

Divide by 100
When we divide by 100, we move the decimal point 2 places to the **left.** This makes the number 100 times smaller.

Divide by 1000
When we divide by 1000, we move the decimal point 3 places to the **left.** This makes the number 1000 times smaller.

$$\frac{X}{Y} = \frac{\text{numerator} = \text{no. of parts used}}{\text{total no. of parts in a whole}}$$

Equivalent fractions **are different ways of writing the same fraction.**
Simplifying fractions – **putting fractions in their simplest form, also known as** cancelling.

For example: Find the biggest number that will divide into the top (numerator) and bottom (denominator) numbers.

$$\frac{8}{24} = \frac{\div 8}{\div 8} = \frac{1}{3}$$

Percentage - A percentage is the same as a fraction out of a 100.
10 % means '10 out of 100' and we often say '10 per cent'
(Cent comes from the Latin word for 100).

fraction to percentage = fraction x 100%

percentage to fraction = percentage ÷ 100 ...then simplify if possible

CHAPTER 3

Common metric unit of measurements – drug dosages

In order to remember the relative value between the units you must place in the logical sequence:-

Gram (g)   =   One letter
Milligram (mg)   =   Two letters
Microgram (mcg) =   Three letters

The following diagram shows you how to convert gram to milligram to microgram and vice versa: -

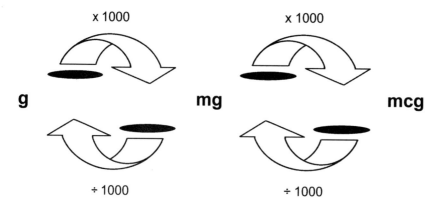

g   **mg**   **mcg**

CHAPTER 4

Common metric unit of measurements – volume

The following diagram shows you how to convert litre to millilitre and vice versa:-

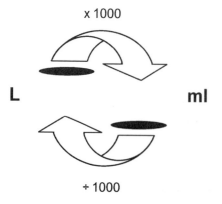

L   **ml**

CHAPTER 5

Calculation of drug dosages:

$$\frac{\text{Prescribed dose (mg) x dilution (ml)}}{\text{Available dose (mg)}}$$

CHAPTER 6

Different infusion sets deliver different amount of fluid (drops) in a ml.

For example: -

20 drops in 1 ml (fluids)
15 drops in 1 ml (blood)
60 mini-drops in 1 ml (for neonatal and young children)

CHAPTER 7

% Concentrations is the amount of drugs dissolved in 100 ml of solution.

For example: -
0.9% of Normal Saline means that there are 0.9 g of Sodium Chloride dissolved in 100 ml of solution.

$$\text{Flow rate (drops/min.)} = \frac{\text{Total volume of fluid (ml) x calibration (drops/ml)}}{\text{Total infusion time (no. of hours x 60 (min.)}}$$

CHAPTER 8

Ratios
For example: -
1 in 1000 means
1 g in 1000 ml of solution = 1000 mg in 1000 ml of solution
= 1 mg in 1 ml

Percentage Volume
0.9% means 9g in 100ml of solution or 900mg in 100ml or 9g in 1000ml

CHAPTER 9

Calculation of paediatric doses: -

Total dose per day =   Child's weight in (kg) x recommended dose of drug (mg) per kg of body weight per day

The calculation for the size of a single dose = $\dfrac{\text{Total dosage per day}}{\text{No. of times per day}}$

CHAPTER 10

Calculation of rate setting for a syringe driver

$$\text{Set Rate} = \dfrac{\textbf{Fluid length in mm}}{\textbf{Infusion time in hours}}$$

CHAPTER 11

Understand the law when dealing with medications.

Understand nurses' responsibilities in accordance with the NMC Document Standards for the Administration of Medicines.

CHAPTER 12

Understand why tablets should not be crushed and capsules should not be opened. Avoid common confusions of medications with very similar names.

CHAPTER 13

The mean is the average of a set of data, obtained by adding together all scores and dividing by the number of data. The median is the middle number of a set of data. The mode is the most frequently occurring number of a set of data.

SUGGESTED READING LISTS AND WEBSITES

Useful Websites

- ❖ http://www.testandcalc.com

- ❖ http://learntech.uwe.ac.uk/numeracy/

- ❖ http://www.lanpdc.scot.nhs.uk/calculations

SUGGESTED READING

White, R. and Bradnam, V (2007) – Handbook of Drug Administration via Enteral Feeding Tubes – London: Pharmaceutical Press.

ANSWERS

Chapter One: Converting pounds to kilograms, and kilograms to pounds

Exercise 1:

1) 2 kg	2) 9 kg	3) 23 kg	4) 6 kg	5) 3 kg
6) 15 kg	7) 60 kg	8) 40 kg	9) 5 kg	10) 7 kg
11) 8.8 lb	12) 4.4 lb	13) 12.1 lb	14) 13.64 lb	15) 16.72 lb
16) 22 lb	17) 99 lb	18) 19.36 lb	19) 77 lb	20) 24.42

Chapter Two : Converting decimals

Exercise 1 :

1) 3.5	2) 71	3) 200	4) 9.9	5) 52
6) 1200	7) 46	8) 850	9) 6700	10) 46.17238
11) 160	12) 3.2	13) 280	14) 6800	15) 7.8
16) 1330	17) 147	18) 5.5	19) 0.18	20) 34
21) 2.12	22) 725	23) 140	24) 2.95	25) 1.78
26) 8812	27) 6012	28) 0.41	29) 672	30) 90.1
31) 90	32) 87.01	33) 100.1	34) 8.05	35) 990
36) 6670	37) 505.1	38) 109.9	39) 801.1	40) 9911

Exercise 2 :

1) 0.07	2) 0.0062	3) 0.0095	4) 0.00011	5) 0.000078
6) 0.0145	7) 1.07	8) 0.10056	9) 0.5673	10) 0.7012
11) 7.538	12) 0.00068	13) 1.58	14) 0.087	15) 0.0045
16) 0.00078	17) 0.059	18) 4.26	19) 1.885	20) 0.0179
21) 0.009	22) 0.0071	23) 0.0091	24) 9.931	25) 0.8031
26) 0.09951	27) 10.11	28) 6.691	29) 1.0101	30) 8.761
31) 9.911	32) 0.413	33) 0.08341	34) 0.6011	35) 7.305
36) 0.0951	37) 4.431	38) 0.0691	39) 34.01	40) 0.09109

Exercise 3:

1) 2, 9, 4, 15, 6	2) 10, 3, 20, 5, 30	3) 2, 24, 4, 40, 6
4) 14, 3, 28, 5, 42	5) 2, 27, 4, 45, 6	

Exercise 4:

1) $\frac{1}{2}$	2) $\frac{1}{5}$	3) $\frac{1}{4}$	4) $\frac{1}{9}$	5) $\frac{6}{7}$	6) $\frac{1}{2}$	7) $\frac{1}{4}$
8) $\frac{1}{8}$	9) $\frac{2}{3}$	10) $\frac{1}{7}$	11) $\frac{3}{4}$	12) $\frac{1}{5}$	13) $\frac{3}{4}$	14) $\frac{2}{7}$
15) $\frac{5}{6}$	16) $\frac{4}{5}$	17) $\frac{1}{4}$	18) $\frac{12}{21} = \frac{4}{7}$	19) $\frac{6}{13}$	20) $\frac{1}{3}$	21) $\frac{1}{2}$
22) $\frac{1}{3}$	23) $\frac{2}{7}$	24) $\frac{2}{7}$	25) $\frac{12}{27} = \frac{4}{9}$	26) $\frac{1}{3}$	27) $\frac{1}{13}$	28) $\frac{1}{4}$
29) $\frac{9}{10}$	30) $\frac{2}{11}$	31) $\frac{4}{5}$	32) $\frac{2}{19}$	33) $\frac{1}{4}$	34) $\frac{6}{7}$	35) $\frac{1}{15}$
36) $\frac{6}{11}$	37) $\frac{4}{27}$	38) $\frac{29}{46}$	39) $\frac{5}{9}$	40) $\frac{1}{3}$		

Exercise 5:

1) 1 2) $2\frac{1}{2}$ 3) $\frac{4}{7}$ 4) $1\frac{1}{5}$ 5) $\frac{1}{3}$ 6) $4\frac{2}{3}$ 7) 3

8) $2\frac{1}{2}$ 9) $2\frac{4}{7}$ 10) $\frac{8}{9}$ 11) $1\frac{1}{2}$ 12) $1\frac{2}{7}$ 13) $1\frac{1}{2}$ 14) $2\frac{5}{8}$

15) $1\frac{13}{14}$ 16) 2 17) $\frac{17}{9} = 1\frac{8}{9}$ 18) $3\frac{3}{7}$ 19) $4\frac{2}{3}$ 20) $3\frac{3}{5}$ 21) $3\frac{4}{7}$

22) $7\frac{1}{2}$ 23) $1\frac{1}{14}$ 24) $2\frac{13}{21}$ 25) $5\frac{5}{9}$ 26) $3\frac{3}{7}$ 27) $4\frac{2}{3}$ 28) $\frac{15}{29}$

29) $\frac{9}{11}$ 30) $1\frac{5}{9}$ 31) $4\frac{9}{10}$ 32) $3\frac{11}{15}$ 33) $\frac{14}{19}$ 34) $3\frac{1}{2}$ 35) 4

36) $1\frac{1}{3}$ 37) $2\frac{5}{11}$ 38) $2\frac{4}{7}$ 39) $3\frac{3}{5}$ 40) $4\frac{1}{5}$

Exercise 6:

1) $2\frac{1}{4}$ 2) $4\frac{1}{4}$ 3) $6\frac{1}{6}$ 4) $5\frac{3}{10}$ 5) $9\frac{7}{9}$ 6) $4\frac{1}{2}$ 7) $3\frac{3}{4}$

8) $15\frac{1}{6}$ 9) $4\frac{9}{10}$ 10) $3\frac{1}{2}$ 11) $11\frac{3}{8}$ 12) $6\frac{3}{4}$ 13) $13\frac{2}{3}$ 14) $11\frac{6}{7}$

15) $25\frac{2}{5}$ 16) $5\frac{1}{8}$ 17) $13\frac{2}{5}$ 18) $10\frac{5}{11}$ 19) $2\frac{1}{2}$ 20) $3\frac{2}{5}$ 21) $15\frac{2}{5}$

22) $1\frac{1}{4}$ 23) 8 24) $1\frac{2}{3}$ 25) $16\frac{1}{2}$ 26) 6 27) $6\frac{2}{15}$ 28) $4\frac{2}{3}$

29) $6\frac{1}{2}$ 30) $1\frac{1}{14}$ 31) $1\frac{1}{2}$ 32) $12\frac{5}{6}$ 33) $2\frac{1}{2}$ 34) $1\frac{5}{9}$ 34) $1\frac{5}{9}$

35) $1\frac{5}{22}$ 36) $1\frac{3}{4}$ 37) $1\frac{6}{7}$ 38) $1\frac{2}{3}$ 39) $1\frac{10}{27}$ 40) $22\frac{1}{3}$

Exercise 7:

1) $\frac{3}{4}$ 2) $\frac{1}{2}$ 3) $\frac{1}{2}$ 4) $\frac{1}{5}$ 5) $\frac{3}{4}$ 6) $1\frac{1}{3}$ 7) $\frac{2}{7}$

8) 4 9) $\frac{5}{6}$ 10) $1\frac{1}{4}$ 11) $\frac{1}{4}$ 12) $\frac{12}{21} = \frac{4}{7}$ 13) $2\frac{1}{6}$ 14) $\frac{1}{3}$

15) $\frac{1}{2}$ 16) $\frac{1}{3}$ 17) $3\frac{1}{2}$ 18) $\frac{2}{7}$ 19) $\frac{1}{2}$ 20) $\frac{4}{9}$

Exercise 8:

1) 5% 2) 10% 3) 4% 4) 20% 5) 50% 6) 40% 7) 25%

8) 100% 9) 10% 10) 20% 11) 150% 12) 75% 13) 200% 14) 80%

15) 300% 16) 30% 17) 15% 18) 16% 19) 8% 20) 20%

Exercise 9:

1) $\frac{13}{100}$ 2) $\frac{31}{50}$ 3) $\frac{1}{20}$ 4) $\frac{71}{100}$ 5) $\frac{13}{50}$ 6) $\frac{39}{50}$ 7) $\frac{9}{100}$

8) $\frac{12}{25}$ 9) $3\frac{33}{100}$ 10) $\frac{97}{100}$ 11) $\frac{21}{100}$ 12) $2\frac{1}{100}$ 13) $\frac{41}{100}$ 14) $1\frac{2}{25}$

15) $\frac{11}{20}$ 16) $\frac{93}{100}$ 17) $\frac{14}{25}$ 18) $\frac{4}{25}$ 19) $1\frac{1}{10}$ 20) $\frac{21}{25}$

Exercise 10:

1) x = 140 2) x = 55 3) x = 36 4) x = 21.6 5) x = 144

6) x = 18.2 7) x = 12 8) x = 87.5 9) x = 4.3 10) x = 22.5

Exercise 11

Fill in the missing blanks:

	Fraction	Ratio	Percentage	Decimal
1)	$\frac{3}{4}$	3:4	75%	0.75
2)	$\frac{1}{2}$	1:2	50%	0.5
3)	$\frac{3}{8}$	3:8	37.5%	0.375
4)	$\frac{11}{20}$	11:20	55%	0.55
5)	$\frac{6}{8}$	6:8	75%	0.75
6)	$\frac{1}{4}$	1:4	25%	0.25
7)	$\frac{1}{8}$	1:8	12.5%	0.125
8)	$\frac{4}{10}$	4:10	40%	0.4
9)	$\frac{1}{5}$	1:5	20%	0.2
10)	$\frac{2}{3}$	2:3	66.6%	0.66
11)	$\frac{16}{100}$	16:100	16%	0.16
12)	$\frac{8}{100}$	8:100	8%	0.8
13)	$\frac{9}{10}$	9:10	90%	0.9
14)	$\frac{1}{3}$	1:3	33.3%	0.33
15)	$\frac{1}{1}$	1:1	100%	1.0
16)	$\frac{7}{10}$	7:10	70%	0.7
17)	$\frac{3}{5}$	3:5	60%	0.6
18)	$\frac{1}{10}$	1:10	10%	0.1
19)	$\frac{9}{20}$	9:20	45%	0.45
20)	$\frac{1}{100}$	1:100	1%	0.01

Chapter Three: Conversion of metric unit weight

Exercise 1:

1) 62.5 mcg	2) 0.5 mg	3) 0.125 mg	4) 250 mcg	5) 0.1 mg
6) 0.15 mg	7) 2000 mcg	8) 0.2 mg	9) 0.025 mg	10) 4000 mcg
11) 3000 mcg	12) 400 mcg	13) 0.5 mg	14) 500000 mcg	15) 2500 mg
16) 0.5 g	17) 0.02 mg	18) 1500 mg	19) 0.5 mg	20) 10 mcg
21) 5 mcg	22) 600 mg	23) 400 mg	24) 50 mcg	

Chapter Four: Conversion of metric unit volume

Exercise 1:

1) 0.25 L	2) 1500 ml	3) 850 ml	4) 0.0245 ml	5) 2750 L
6) 0.75 L	7) 25 ml	8) 0.023 L	9) 0.0285 L	10) 0.0075 L
11) 0.0091 L	12) 0.225 L	13) 150 ml	14) 20 ml	15) 0.505 L
16) 0.0425 L	17) 1008 ml	18) 0.35 L	19) 9 ml	20) 2250 ml

Chapter Five : Calculating drug dosage

Exercise 1:

1) 1.2 5 ml	2) 8.75 ml	3) 20 ml	4) 4 ml	5) 10 ml
6) 1.25 ml	7) 1½ tablets	8) 7.5 ml	9) 2.5 ml	10) 15 ml
11) 7.5 ml	12) 1.25 ml	13) 2 ml	14) 2.5 ml	15) 1.5 ml
16) 16 ml	17) 10 ml	18) 17 ml	19) 1.6 ml	20) 15ml
21) 5 ml	22) 0.2 ml	23) 1.33 ml	24) 4 ml	25) 5 ml
26) 1.5 ml	27) 15 ml	28) 20 ml	29) 3 tablets	30) 10 ml

Chapter Six: Calculating fluids

Exercise 1:

1) 83.33 drops/min	2) 55.5 drops/min.	3) 33.33 drops/min.
4) 41.66 drops/min.	5) 27.77 drops/min.	6) 13.88 drops/min.
7) 27.77 drops/min.	8) 66.66 drops/min.	9) 33.33/min.
10) 55.55 drops/min.		

Exercise 2:

1) 28.125 drops/min.	2) 20.83 drops/min.	3) 41.66 drops/min.
4) 25 drops/min.	5) 20.83 drops/min.	6) 21.87 drops/min.
7) 18.75 drops/min.	8) 31.25 drops/min.	9) 37.5 drops/min.
10) 31.25 drops/min.		

Exercise 3:

1) 83.3 drops/min	2) 41.66 drops/min.	3) 62.5 drops/min.
4) 50 drops/min.	5) 75 drops/min	6) 80 drops/min.
7) 40 drops/min.	8) 55.5 drops/min.	9) 70 drops/min
10) 90 drops/min.		

Exercise 4:

1) 100ml/hr	2) 125 ml/hr	3) 125 ml/hr	4) 83.33 ml/hr
5) 166.66 ml/hr	6) 200 ml/hr	7) 111.11 ml/hr	8) 90.9 drops/hr
9) 100ml/hr	10) 166.66 ml/hr		

Chapter Seven : Calculation of I.V.flow rate for I.V.drug dosages

Exercise 1:

1a) 60 drops	1b) 20 drops	2a) 30 drops
2b) 10 drops	3a) 240 drops	3b) 80 drops
4a) 120 drops	4b) 40 drops	5a) 120 drops
5b) 40 drops	6a) 72 drops	6b) 24 drops
7a) 30 mg	7b) 60 drops	8a) 40 mcg
8b) 24 drops	9) 100 mg	9b) 80 drops
10a) 600 mcg or 0.6 mg	10b) 18 drops	11a) 50 mg
11b) 10 ml	12a) 25 mg	12b) 12.5 ml
13a) 24000 mcg or 24 mg	13b) 2.4 ml	14a) 125 mg
14b) 25 ml	15a) 1500 mg or 1.5 g	15b) 15 ml
16a) 60 mg	16b) 4 ml	17a) 3000 mcg or 3 mg
17b) 0.75 ml	18a) 5000 mcg or 5 mg	18b) 2.5 ml
19a) 50 mg	19b) 25 ml	20a) 9000 mcg or 9 mg
20b) 0.9 ml		

Chapter Eight : Ratios and percentages

Exercise 1

1) 1 mg in 200ml	2) 1 mg in 80 ml	3) 1 mg in 5 ml	4) 10 mg in 1 ml
5) 1mg in 10ml	6) 1mg in 20 ml	7) 1 mg in 50 ml	8) 1 mg in 8 ml
9) 1 mg in 4 ml	10) 1 mg in 60 ml		

Exercise 2

1) 100 mg	2) 40 mg	3) 1000 mg	4) 100 mg	5) 900 mg
6) 1800 mg	7) 2500 mg	8) 4000 mg	9) 1000 mg	10) 10 mg
11) 1250 mg	12) 2500 mg	13) 3000 mg	14) 380 mg	15) 2800 mg
16) 2500 mg	17) 450 mg	18) 1000 mg	19) 1500 mg	20) 6000 mg

Exercise 3

1) 5 g or 5000 mg in 100ml	2) 0.45 g or 450 mg in 100 ml
3) 0.225 g or 225 mg in 100 ml	4) 0.18 g or 180 mg in 100 ml
5) 4 g or 4000 mg in 100 ml	6) 10 g or 10,000 mg in 100 ml
7) 2.5 g or 2500 mg in 100 ml	8) 6 g or 6000 mg in 100 ml
9) 3.86 g or 3860 mg in 100 ml	10) 0.2 g or 200 mg in 100 ml
11) 0.1 g or 100 mg in 100 ml	12) 0.15 g or 150 mg in 100 ml
13) 0.05 g or 50 mg in 100 ml	14) 0.001 g or 1 mg in 100 ml
15) 0.375 g or 375 mg in 100 ml	16) 0.44 g or 440 mg in 100 ml
17) 0.12 g or 120 mg in 100 ml	18) 0.025 g or 25 mg in 100 ml
19) 0.035 g or 35 mg in 100 ml	20) 0.0075 g or 7.5 mg in 100

Exercise 4

1) 20%	2) 5%	3) 30%	4) 20%	5) 0.1%
6) 1.5%	7) 2%	8) 10%	9) 0.2 %	10) 2.5%
11) 0.1%	12) 1 %	13) 0.05 %	14) 0.4 %	15) 0.005%
16) 5%	17) 2.4%	18) 10%	19) 0.8%	20) 5 %

Chapter Nine : Calculating paediatric doses

Exercise 1:

1a) 800 mg/day   1b) 200 mg/single dose   2a) 800 mg/day
2b) 200 mg/single dose   3a) 45 mg/day   3b) 15 mg/single dose
4a) 750 mg/day   4b) 187.5 mg/dose   5) 5000 mcg/day or 5 mg/day
6a) 15mg/day   6b) 7.5 mg/single dose   7a) 250 mg/day
7b) 125 mg/single dose   8a) 300 mg/day   8b) 100 mg/single dose
9a) 400 mg/day   9b) 100 mg/single dose   10a) 40 mg/day
10b) 20 mg/single dose

Exercise 2 :

1) 3 ml	2) 0.6 ml	3) 8 ml	4) 0.83 ml	5) 4 ml
6) 0.7 ml	7) 1.6 ml	8) 0.25 ml	9) 12 ml	10) 0.6 ml
11) 2 tablets	12) 8 ml	13) 15 ml	14) 6 ml	15) 2.5 ml
16) 12.5 ml	17) 0.25 ml	18) 7.5 ml	19) 7.5 ml	20) 4 ml

INDEX

Answers 86

Arithmetic mean 77

Calculating drug dosages 35

       drug dosages in children 57

       drug flow rates 47

       infusion flow rates 41

       intravenous fluids 41

Calibration 41

Calculating dosages for syringe drivers 63

Centimetres 1

Child body weight 57

Common factors 17

Controlled Drugs 67,70

Converting ....

       decimals 5

       fractions into percentages 18

       improper fractions into mixed fractions 16

       kilograms into pounds 3

       litres to millilitres 31

       metric units of weight 25

       millilitres to litres 31

       pounds into kilograms 3

       the ratio and percentages of drugs 53

Crushing tablets 73

Decimalisation 2

Decimals 5

Denominator 10, 11, 12, 16, 17

Descriptive statistics 77

Distance 1,2

Divide 5

Dosages 2, 3

Drops per minute 41

Drug concentration 54

Drug dose 35

Enteric coated 74

Equivalent fractions 12

Extremes 21

Flow rates 41

Fluid length 65

Foot 1

Formula 35

Fractions 5, 10, 11, 15

Frequency 79

g 2, 3

Gallon 1

General Sales List 69

Gram 1, 2, 4

Histogram 79

Hundredweight 1

Imperial 2, 3

Imperial System 1

Improper fractions 5, 16, 17

Inch 1

Infusion time 65

Intravenous fluids 41

Kg 2, 3, 4

Kilo 2

Kilogram 1, 2, 3, 4

Kilometre 1, 4

Km 2

L 2

Law 67

lb 3

Legal classification of drugs 67

Litres .... 1, 2, 4 mcg 3

Mean 21, 77

Measures of central tendency 77

Median 77

Medicine classifications 69

Medicines Act 1971 69

Metres 1, 2, 4

Metric System 1, 3

Metric Units 2

mg 2, 3

Microgram 3

Mile 1, 2

Milli 2

Milligram 1, 2, 3, 4

Millilitres 1, 2

Millilitres per hour 41

Millimetres 1, 2

Misuse of drugs act 1971 67

Mixed fractions 5, 15, 16

ml 2

Modal value 79

Mode 77

Modified release 74

Multiplication ....

       of a fraction by a whole number 14

       of fractions 14

       of a decimal 6

Multiply 5

Numerator 10, 11, 12, 16,17

Ounce 1, 3

Oz 3

Paediatric drug doses 57

Percentage 5, 18

Percentage concentration 54

Percentages 53

Pharmacy Only 70

Pint 1

Pounds 1, 3, 4

Prescription Only Medicine 70

Prescriptions 2

Product 21

Proportion 20, 22

Quart 1

Ratios and percentages 53

Ratios 5, 20, 22, 53

Reference section 80

Routes of administration 71

S.I. Units 1

Schedules of controlled drugs 67, 68

Set rate 65

Statistics 77

Stone 1

Suggested reading 85

        websites 85

Symbol 1, 3

Syringe driver 63

Unit of time 41

Units 1

Units of measurement 1

Volume 1, 2

Weight 1, 2, 3

Yard 1

¼ 3